The Diabetic's Total Health Book

REVISED AND EXPANDED

Also by June Biermann and Barbara Toohey

The Woman's Holistic Headache Relief Book

The Diabetic's Sports and Exercise Book

The Diabetic's Book: All Your Questions Answered

The Peripatetic Diabetic

The Diabetic Woman
(with Lois Jovanovic, M.D.)

The Diabetic Man
(with Peter Lodewick, M.D.)

Under the name Margaret Bennett

Biking for Grownups

Cross-Country Skiing for the Fun of It

How to Ski Just a Little Bit

Dr. Owl's Problem

From Baedeker to Worse

Alice in Womanland

THE THIRD REVISED EDITION

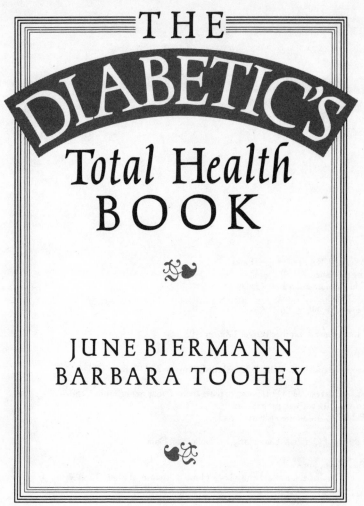

THE DIABETIC'S Total Health BOOK

JUNE BIERMANN
BARBARA TOOHEY

Foreword by Fred Whitehouse, M.D.
Past President of the American Diabetes Association

Jeremy P. Tarcher/Perigee

Jeremy P. Tarcher/Perigee Books
are published by
The Putnam Publishing Group
200 Madison Avenue
New York, NY 10016

First Jeremy P. Tarcher/Perigee Edition 1992

Library of Congress Cataloging-in-Publication Data

Biermann, June.
The diabetic's total health book / June Biermann, Barbara Toohey.
—3rd rev. ed.
p. cm.
Includes bibliographical references and index.
ISBN 0-87477-689-9
1. Diabetes. 2. Health. 3. Diabetes—Diet therapy—Recipes.
I. Toohey, Barbara. II. Title.
RC660.B47 1992
616.4'62—dc20 92-7076 CIP

Printed in the United States of America
2 3 4 5 6 7 8 9 10

This book is printed on acid-free paper.

To Betty Annis
for years and years and years
of total love,
encouragement, and support.

Contents

Foreword

"Our remedies oft in ourselves do lie."
—Shakespeare,
All's Well That Ends Well, I, i, 231

This is a lovely book. It expresses a "can do" attitude. We learn why people with diabetes should actively participate in their own medical care. The authors remind us how well a diabetic person feels when the diabetes stays controlled. We come to understand that no obstacle is totally insurmountable. Prudent eating habits, sports, and exercise, and a positive mental outlook, as well as more innovative techniques like laughter and hug therapy, become integral parts of total health.

Fostering these active-positive attitudes adds to the quality of life whether or not one has diabetes. Stress lessens and optimism flowers. Good self-care is accentuated.

This book discusses many agreeable activities, and yet the authors suggest that not every activity, no matter how beneficial it may seem, is necessarily the proper choice for every individual. They wisely point out the possible options so that we can make personal choices.

As I read this book, random thoughts surfaced. Let me share a couple with you.

"Control your diabetes to live; don't live to control your diabetes." *Keep your priorities in proper order.*

"Surely the whole person is greater than the sum of the parts." *Don't talk to me about a diabetic; talk to me about a person with diabetes.*

Savor this book; it is vintage Biermann-Toohey. They have used diabetes as a role model for coping with life. They have shown us how simple living and thinking will embellish a lifestyle. Since they themselves are compleat people, we should consider their views and find ways to incorporate those thoughts and activities that we find personally compatible. Here is a book that makes us think. Surely, this is the mark of something new that is worthwhile.

FRED WHITEHOUSE, M.D.
Chief, Division of Endocrinology and Metabolism
Henry Ford Hospital
Detroit, Michigan
Past President, American Diabetes Association

Preface

We're delighted to have the opportunity to write this second revision of *The Diabetic's Total Health Book.* So many beneficial changes have taken place in the three years since the first revision that the world of total health for diabetics is now a new and better place and we are now new—and we hope better!—people. This edition incorporates these changes. We urge you to add them, along with our other basic principles of total health, to your way of life and thereby create a new and better you.

HEAD START

Twenty-five years ago, when the June half of our writing collaboration first discovered she had diabetes, we were determined that she wasn't going to roll over and play disabled. We set out to find ways for her to continue to lead her active and exciting life. Using our research training as college librarians, and with June as a willing guinea pig for our experiments, we succeeded beyond our most optimistic expectations.

We spread the encouraging word of our discoveries in our book *The Peripatetic Diabetic.* In our talks before diabetes groups and in letters we received from diabetics we picked up more life-enhancing ideas. We reported these, along with our own continuing living and learning experiences, in more books and in articles in *Diabetes Forecast* and *Diabetes in the News.*

Then June, whom we call "the woman who has everything," developed another health problem—intense and incapacitating chronic headaches. These had nothing to do with her diabetes, but it took us five years of research and experimentation to find out what they did have to do with and how to cure them.

During this long, painful search for relief from headaches, June serendipitously discovered a different approach to life and health—and to diabetes control. This new and yet ancient approach goes by a now passé buzzword, holism, but we prefer to think of it simply as a way of living that results in total health of body, mind, and spirit.

Although you may not be aware of it, as a diabetic you are no stranger to these total-health practices. You're already familiar with one of the essential ideas—the idea that *you* are the person responsible for keeping yourself well. Isn't that what your doctor told you when you were first diagnosed diabetic? Weren't you told that you had to master the diet and stick to it, get your exercise, inject your insulin or swallow your pills, check your blood sugar regularly, and that your doctor couldn't do any of these things for you? With this little lecture you got your first lesson in self-responsibility as a necessary component of total health.

THE WHOLE STORY OF CONTROL

Another important concept, one you may be only peripherally aware of, is that everything about you is involved with your health and, hence, everything about you—not just your islets of Langerhans—is involved with your diabetes. What you eat, drink, and breathe; your physical activity; your emotions; your sleep and rest; your work; your natural and social environment; your lifestyle—every aspect of your life profoundly affects the level of your blood sugar. The holistic or total-health approach recognizes this interconnectedness and helps you work toward seeing yourself as a whole ("holism" is sometimes spelled "wholism") and treating yourself accordingly.

When speaking before diabetes groups we've been asked more than once by some member of the audience, "Why, when I eat exactly the same lunch two days in a row, do I sometimes have high blood sugar one day and low or normal the next?" The answer is simply that one or more of the multitudinous interconnected variables of your body-mind-emotion-environment complex was different the second day. You cannot control your diabetes by the diet factor alone, nor by any other isolated factor. You always have to consider your wholeness, your totality.

Notice that we are saying *your* wholeness, *your* totality because, besides being all wrapped up in one package, you are a unique package. Your particular collection of living cells is different in many ways from any other collection. For that reason the way you take care of your health and your diabetes must be tailored to you, not to some standardized prototype diabetic.

The rationale behind this philosophy of individualism in treatment is beginning to emerge from the scientific community. Diabetes is now being recognized as not resulting solely from a pancreas that is not making enough insulin but from a variety of causes. Actually only about 15 percent of diabetics don't produce enough insulin. The rest have a problem with getting their insulin into the cells—and even that problem has more than one cause.

PREVENTIVE MAINTENANCE

At this point, you may be asking yourself what your doctor's contribution is to this very individual treatment for this very individual diabetic. Since self-analysis and self-responsibility are such a big part of total health, did June just take over her diabetes, stop going to her doctor, and forget all the advances medical science has made in diabetes care? Not on your life (or hers)! June works more closely than ever with her doctor. The two of them are total partners in the maintenance of her total health.

The maintenance-of-health aspect is particularly important. The basic idea is that you work with your doctor to keep well. You don't let yourself fall apart and then run to your doctor to get glued together again. Your doctor will no doubt vastly prefer helping you maintain good health rather than trying to repair the possibly irreparable damages you can cause by ignorance, indifference, or indolence.

IN SICKNESS AND IN HEALTH

We once heard a doctor make an interesting distinction between disease and health. He said you can be completely free from disease and yet be unhealthy—run down, flabby, sallow, sluggish, unproductive, depressed; or, in other words, a physical, mental, and emotional mess. On the other hand, you can have a definite chronic illness like diabetes and yet be healthy—strong, lithe, lean, vigorous, alert, productive, and enthusiastic; or, in other words, a physical, mental, and emotional triumph.

We want to help you achieve this kind of triumph by helping you change your outlook. Instead of focusing on your disease, begin focusing on your health. Think of yourself as making changes in your lifestyle not because you're a diabetic but because you want to be a healthy, happy, productive person. The changes we're recommending are not restrictive; they are expansive. They are the kinds of changes that every person who wants to enjoy life to the fullest should be making—and many are. Barbara, the nondiabetic half of the collaboration, willingly—even *eagerly*—follows exactly the regime we suggest for a diet-controlled diabetic.

THE SCHOOL OF HARD KNOCKS

In retrospect, June feels it was worthwhile to suffer through those five years of headache pain because it provided such a tremendous learning experience. As Flannery O'Connor has said, "Sickness is a place more instructive than a long trip to Europe." The changes June learned to make in her life because of her headaches have, indeed, given her increased mastery over diabetes; but what is even more important is that they have brought about the kind of overall physical, mental, emotional, and spiritual transformation that makes for a productive and happy life—a life in which every year you live seems like the best.

We hope that this book will do painlessly for you what June's headaches did for her.

INTRODUCTION

Stress and the Diabetic

THE DIABETES POPULATION BOMB

Here are some discouraging statistics from a 1991 American Diabetes Association news release: "In a 1990 report, the Centers for Disease Control stated the diabetes incidence rate increased 17 percent between 1980 and 1987, rising from an estimated 6 million to an estimated 7 million Americans. However, the CDC notes that since about half of all diabetes cases are unreported, the true incidence of the disease may be some 14 million persons."

If this trend continues and no cure is found, on some future someday everyone in the country will be diabetic. While this should make it easier to get a piece of fruit for dessert in a restaurant, it has few other pleasant dividends.

Why this big upturn in diabetes? Dr. O. Charles Olson, former director of the Diabetes Education Center of the Deaconess Hospital in Spokane, Washington, explains it this way: "First of all, Americans eat too much and generally are too fat. Next, Americans are living longer, and since many people are now entering and living through the 65- to 74-year span (the ages of the greatest incidence of inception of diabetes), many of them are developing diabetes. Modern diagnostic methods and the awareness of the public to the need for good medical care results in diagnosing diabetes oftener and sooner."

PUBLIC ENEMY NUMBER ONE

While all of this is certainly true, we don't believe it is the whole answer to the burgeoning diabetes population. As they say about the disease, heredity loads the gun but something else pulls the trigger. We are convinced that the most trigger-happy something else in modern America is stress. There is, in fact, an increasing realization among health professionals that the pressures and tensions and pollutions of our daily lives underlie most of our major chronic health problems: arthritis, cardiovascular disease, respiratory disease, cancer—and diabetes.

It has long been known that in those people with the genetic tendency toward the disease, diabetes can be brought on by stress—by the physical stress of pregnancy, an automobile accident, surgery, or overweight; or by the emotional stress of something like a death in the family, a divorce, or the loss of a job. What has been ignored is the fact that stress's dirty work does not end there. Stress can also be the ruination of diabetes control on a day-to-day basis. Even worse, as Drs. David S. Schade and R. Philip Eaton reported in the November 30, 1979, issue of *Journal of the American Medical Association,* "The most common precipitating cause of ketoacidosis [the diabetic state that can lead to coma and death] is not omission of insulin but the presence of a stress." However, no one seems to be delivering the messages clearly to diabetics or doing anything much about giving them the tools for stress management.

The first major diabetes teaching program to give systematic instruction in stress-lowering techniques was the one at the Kansas Regional Diabetes Center in Wichita. Diana Guthrie, the Center's diabetes nurse specialist and the recipient of an Ames Award as the outstanding nonphysician health-care educator of the year told us that they did a study using biofeedback to teach relaxation to diabetics with special problems like alcoholism and overweight. The results proved that "learning to manage stress really does cause stabilization and lowering of blood sugar." As a result they incorporated several self-help therapies for stress reduction into their teaching program for all diabetics, and teaching programs all across the nation have followed suit.

But as so often happens in matters of diabetes care, astute diabetics have often had to figure out for themselves that control is strongly affected by stress levels. For example, we once wrote a column in *Diabetes in the News* about those aspects of diabetes that irritated June the most. We then invited readers to send us their own gripes.

Beverly Meyerheim complained about "the continued lack of recognition . . . of the relationship of blood-sugar levels . . . to the nervous system, brain, emotions, and behavior. Stress therapy and learning new adaptive responses can be most helpful. The instruction to 'tend to your emotions' is not very explicit."

And another diabetic, Dale B. Pierce, after airing some of her complaints, wrote, "If I had any words for young diabetics they would be to avoid as much stress as possible. Sometimes we try to make our bodies do as much as three or four people at once and it shows up in later life."

Some diabetics do try to do "as much as three or four people at once" just to prove that they can, just to prove they are not handicapped in any way. Even we, with our firm belief in the detrimental effects of stress, sometimes fall into this trap. We were once on a two-week book-promotion tour, appearing on radio and TV and flying to a different city each day. It was grueling and exhausting enough to kill a nondiabetic ox. June grew understandably weary and even picked up a case of food poisoning and developed a fever. It looked for a while as if she might not be able to finish the tour. "You've got to go on," Barbara kept saying as she dosed June with vitamin C. "We're always telling people that a diabetic can do *everything.* You don't want to make liars out of us!" June did go on. She never missed a show.

At the end of the tour in Boston we called on the famous diabetologist Dr. Priscilla White, who had recently retired from Boston's famed Joslin Clinic. When we related this story to her with a certain amount of pride of accomplishment, Dr. White smiled wisely. "Yes, I agree," she said. "A diabetic *can* do everything. But a diabetic doesn't *have to* do everything."

A STRESS WITHIN A STRESS WITHIN A STRESS WITHIN A STRESS

June has always believed that diabetes itself is a tremendous stress factor. The blood-sugar swings provide the physical stress. The worry over the timing of meals, the availability of food, the fitting into your life of diabetic routines such as all the blood sugar testing, and the awkward social problems occasioned by trying to follow your diet when dining out at a restaurant or in someone's home all contribute to emotional tensions, which, in turn, are detrimental to control.

How does stress work to undermine diabetes control? Very simply put, it's this way. Stress activates the adrenal glands to bring about the fight-or-flight response built into our systems in the days when we had to either whap a dinosaur over the head or outrun him. The adrenalin would flow, signaling an increase in blood pressure and heart rate, muscular tension, a rising of blood-cholesterol levels, and, most significant for diabetics, a release of sugar from the liver to give us the fuel for the fight or flight. After the danger was over the adrenals would shut down, allowing our ancient ancestor to relax until the next dinosaur arrived.

Today we don't generally get into literal physical altercations, nor do we do much actual sprinting away from danger. Still, we keep triggering nature's alarm system. Because of a hectic pace, tense work, a boss we're not overly fond of, problems with our spouses, children, or parents, or because of city noises hammering away in our subconscious or financial worries or a million other or's, we tend to live in a constant state of stress. The adrenals seldom shut down and let us relax.

They continually send out the signal to the liver, and up goes the blood sugar.

Stress is hard on everyone, but at least in the case of a nondiabetic the pancreas can jump into the fray and squirt out an extra supply of insulin. An insulin-dependent diabetic has to inject more insulin, which tends to make his or her blood sugar swing from high to low; in the case of a diet- or pill-controlled diabetic, the stress may perhaps require insulin injections.

One young adult diabetic, who originally controlled his disease with pills, told us that when he was in college he was cramming a year of Japanese study into a six-week session and at the same time was having problems with his wife. Four weeks into this stressful period, he flunked out on the pills and had to go onto thirty units of insulin. That was eight years ago. He has been on insulin ever since.

But the most vivid personal account of how stress can put your diabetes on a roller coaster came to us from Daisy Kuhn, professor of biology at California State University, Northridge. At the end of the college semester when she's reading her students' masters theses under the pressure of the commencement-ceremony deadline, her insulin dosage is thirty-eight units and she must omit her usual bedtime snack. Still, she wakes up in the morning with high blood sugar. On the other hand, as soon as the semester's over and she's home puttering around, her insulin dosage goes down to thirty-three units, she can have her evening snack again, and she wakes up with normal or even low blood sugar.

One summer Daisy went back to campus to help students applying for medical school. She interviewed them straight through from 1:00 P.M. to 6:00 P.M. When she got home and took her blood sugar on her handy-dandy blood sugar self-testing meter, it was hitting the heights of 330. Later that same week she went to a conference in Asilomar, a beautiful wooded area on the Northern California coast a few miles south of Monterey. After the conference she took the weekend off just to rest and enjoy the scenery. She passed out from low blood sugar.

Daisy told us that when she puts herself under pressure by "turning on the steam," even though she's enjoying the work and feeling the exhilaration of accomplishment, she either has to forgo eating 450 calories or increase her insulin to cover that amount of calories. In other words, the blood-sugar effect of high stress in her case is almost the equivalent of eating a full meal!

Stress has other unfortunate side effects for diabetics. One diabetic told us that when she's under extreme stress, as she was recently when her husband died in an automobile accident, she just ignores her diabetes. In comparison to the problems she's trying to cope with, the diabetes doesn't seem important.

It is also true that as a result of childhood conditioning many of us seek the comfort of food when we're nervous or upset or under pressure. (A friend of ours put on fifteen pounds when she was studying for the bar exam.) The increased weight causes a diabetic more physical stress—and emotional distress—creating still more diabetic problems, and so the vicious circle spins.

Now, no one living in today's world can eliminate stress entirely. You wouldn't want to even if you could, because, as stress expert Hans Selye says, "Stress is the spice of life." It is even stressful when wonderful things happen to you, which Selye calls "eustress," as opposed to distress. When we went on a tour of the Hawaiian Islands with a group of diabetics, many of them reported that when they were getting ready for the trip they were so happily excited that their diabetes got out of control.

Another point that Selye makes is that stress will cause a body to break down at its weakest point, just as a chain breaks at its weakest link. Your weak point obviously has to do with your body's production and/or use of insulin, so you can expect your diabetes problems to escalate in proportion to your escalating stress level.

RECOGNIZING STRESSORS

To keep your most vulnerable area from breaking down, the first step is to learn how to assess your stressors. In this section we're going to give you some good techniques for analyzing the pressures in your life and for recognizing the body's reaction to them. Many Americans have lived with tension so long that they're totally unaware that they're tied in more knots than a macrame wall hanging. They don't even remember what it feels like to be relaxed.

Life Changes

Any change in your life can bring on stress, whether the change is for better or worse. A normal event that causes you to have to change or adapt to new situations—any alteration in your life that requires you to adjust—is a stressor. If too many changes are made too quickly and too frequently without enough time for recovery, you undergo a damaging stress reaction. In your case this can mean wild blood-sugar fluctuations, and these in turn will break down your physical and psychological defenses so that you develop infections, foot and eye problems, depression, and other dismals of diabetes.

Two researchers at the University of Washington in Seattle, Thomas H. Holmes and Richard H. Rahe, devised a chart and point scale of the stressful life happenings that can bring on or exacerbate illness. To use the chart, check off events that have happened to you within the last year and then total up the score by adding up the assigned values. If your score is 150, you have a fifty-fifty chance of worsening your diabetes and/or developing some other illness. A score of over 300 indicates a 90 percent chance for illness. It's not the individual events but the cluster that causes your resistance to disease to be lowered.

You might find a direct connection between the onset of your diabetes and stress by calculating what your chances of developing an illness were according to this chart the year before you were diagnosed diabetic.

Social Readjustment Rating Scale

EVENT	VALUE
Death of spouse	100
Divorce	73
Marital separation	65
Jail term	63
Death of close family member	63
Personal injury or illness	53
Marriage	50
Fired from work	47
Marital reconciliation	45
Retirement	45
Change in family member's health	44
Pregnancy	40
Sex difficulties	39
Addition to family	39
Business readjustment	39
Change in financial status	38
Death of close friend	37
Change to different line of work	36
Change in number of marital arguments	35
Mortgage or loan over $10,000	31
Foreclosure of mortgage or loan	30
Change in work responsibilities	29
Son or daughter leaving home	29
Trouble with in-laws	29
Outstanding personal achievement	28
Spouse begins or stops work	26
Starting or finishing school	26
Change in living conditions	25
Revision of personal habits	24

Trouble with boss	23
Change in work hours, conditions	20
Change in residence	20
Change in schools	20
Change in recreational habits	19
Change in church activities	19
Change in social activities	18
Mortgage or loan under $10,000	17
Change in sleeping habits	16
Change in number of family gatherings	15
Change in eating habits	15
Vacation	13
Christmas season	12
Minor violation of the law	11

Recently a group of psychiatrists expanded this list of life changes and classified them according to desirable and undesirable. Then they studied thirty-seven diabetics for a year or more and discovered that there was definitely a relationship between the occurrence of life changes and adverse effects on diabetes. More significantly, they found that *undesirable* events, in particular, were the most detrimental for diabetics. In an article in the journal *Diabetes,* Dr. Lawrence E. Hinkle, Jr., of New York Hospital, pointed out that the kinds of undesirable life situations that caused the greatest adverse effect on diabetes control were either "acute conflicts with significant individuals," usually parents, husbands, wives, or children, or the threat of the loss of such a significant person.

Body Language

Besides monitoring your life changes for stress, you can also watch your body patterns. Our bodies give off signals when they're tense. Learn these signals and you'll know when you'd better start doing something about the tightness, tension, and anxiety you're exhibiting.

Breathing. This is the best indicator of what's going on inside you, and is often the very first sign. Short and shallow breathing means tension; holding your breath means extreme tension.

Muscle stiffness and aching. These reflect tightness and gripping over long periods of time. Head, neck, shoulder, and upper back muscles are most involved. When you grip hard you often tighten your fist, hunch your shoulders, or clench your jaw.

Warmth. Overworked nerves create heat; you may even perspire under too much pressure, literally breaking into a sweat.

Fatigue. Anxiety and frustration cause exhaustion, even though you may be doing nothing strenuous physically. Emotion, especially bottled-up emotion, is the problem, not overwork.

BLOCK THAT STRESS

All right, then, what are you to do when you find yourself assailed by too many changes and holding your breath over them? You can't become a hermit or a dropout from life. You have to and *want* to take an active part in the world, no matter how stressful that world is. Naturally, you should try to avoid any stresses that *are* avoidable. You'd no more court stress than you'd court disaster. (For a diabetic they can be the same thing.) Nor would you try to numb out the stress with such destructive drugs as Valium and alcohol. No, for all the stresses that can't be avoided (or that you don't want to avoid) what you must do is find ways—healthful ways—to diminish their adverse effects on you. After all, in most cases it is not external stress that causes your diabetic problems but your internal reaction to this stress. Incidentally, Selye says that different people can tolerate different levels of stress. Those he calls "tortoises" can comfortably handle very little stress. They need tranquillity. Those he designates "hares" thrive on stress levels that would flatten a tortoise. In fact, hares feel stressed if they don't have a certain amount of excitement—thrills and chills—in their lives. (*Note:* tortoises and hares almost invariably marry each other, thereby creating stressful stress capacity conflicts.) But whether you're a tortoise or a hare you have to learn how to keep stress—both physical and mental—from getting to you.

In the pages that follow we'll provide you with the blueprints and tools you need to build three virtually impenetrable barriers to the destructive effects of stress: a strong body, a tranquil mind, and a blithe spirit.

PART I

A Strong Body

What makes for good physical health? Heredity, of course, is a major factor, but it's a little late to select new ancestors if yours have left you with a few holes in your genes, such as your tendency toward diabetes. What counts now is what you do with what you've got: the food and chemicals you do or don't put into your body and the activities you do or don't ask your body to perform.

One surgeon general's report on health promotion and disease prevention laid it on the line, stating that "as many as half of American deaths are attributed to unhealthy behavior or lifestyle." To express these concepts in automotive terms, at birth you may have been given a Rolls Royce or a Hyundai. That you can't change. But you are the one who is responsible for filling with fuel and driving and maintaining the machine you were born with. Whether you have a long lifetime of efficient, carefree transportation from your body or a quick, sputtering trip to the junkyard is up to you.

CHAPTER 1
Self-Control

Although in this book we're emphasizing your health rather than your disease, it's a given that if you're going to pursue stress reduction and optimum health you're going to have to start from a base of good diabetes control. If your diabetes is out of control it's a wretched stress on the body, it opens the door for all kinds of minor and major infections, and it just plain makes you feel rotten—exhausted, listless, and sometimes even nauseated. But that's not the worst part. If you know anything about diabetes, you know that long-term out-of-control blood sugar is what causes the dread complications you always hear about and keep trying to push out of your mind. But they won't be pushed out. The worry is always there when your blood sugars are consistently running high or bouncing all over the map. This makes for a heavy, never-departing, built-in stress, but it's one you can get rid of with good control, because, now hear this, the majority of the leading experts in the field of diabetes now concur that *keeping blood sugar in the normal range will prevent complications.*

That good control, that normal blood sugar, is up to you. Fortunately, for the first time in the history of diabetes, the tools of good control are there. (If you had to go and get diabetes, at least you picked the right time!) At last you can know what your blood sugars are—virtually instantly and virtually painlessly—with a simple test in which you prick your finger, get a small drop of blood, put it on a strip, and read it either in a blood sugar meter or (less accurately) by comparing colors to a chart on the strip container. When you chart your blood sugars, your doctor can work with you toward keeping them in the normal range with insulin or oral medications and/or diet and exercise.

The costs of blood sugar testing are not insignificant, but they're changing for the better (meter cost) and for the worse (strip cost). The meter prices constantly get lower; some are actually free, what with rebates and trade-in offers. Prices range from $50 to $180, depending on the technology. The problem is that there is an almost confusing array of choices—fourteen different ones at the moment—and it's not easy to find a supplier who will show them all to you and explain their pros and cons. Base your choice on the recommendation of your doctor or nurse and on how well you like using that particular model. (If you don't like it, you won't use it!) And above all, be sure that whoever sells it to you gives you thorough instruction in its operation.

Test strips used in meters continue to go up in price. They now run from 52 cents to 70 cents each. You can pay even more if you use certain local pharmacies or if the supplier has to bill your health insurance. Incidentally, almost all insurance companies, realizing that good control keeps you out of the hospital and ultimately saves them money, are at least partially paying for meters and strips. Even Medicare pays a major portion of the cost of meters and strips for insulin-taking diabetics, although Type II diabetics are out of luck until the regulations for qualifying are changed.

The best news is that there will soon be a meter not requiring strips or blood. It operates via a beam of infrared light shined onto the finger.

For insulin-takers there have been a lot of improvements, too, including devices that shoot the needle into you quickly and painlessly: the Inject-Ease, the Injectomatic, the Instaject, and the Autojector. The Autojector also automatically injects the insulin. Then there are jet injectors which have no needle at all. The insulin is injected literally at the speed of a jet—the insulin itself becomes a needle. These jet injectors not only eliminate the trauma of having to stick yourself with a needle but also make for improved insulin absorption, since the insulin doesn't pool at the injection site. The jet injectors currently available are the Medi-Jector II, the Medi-Jector EZ and Tender Touch, the Preci-Jet 50, and the VitaJet II.

Another new injection development is the arrival of penlike devices for injecting small amounts of insulin by clicking or twisting. With these you can inject the number of units you want without having to fill a syringe ahead of time. This is extremely convenient when you're injecting before meals away from home. These devices include the NovoPen and the NovolinPen.

FELLED BY ONE SHOT

The devices we just mentioned for insulin-injection are designed to make it easier and more acceptable for Type I (insulin-dependent) diabetics to take multiple shots of insulin. Multiple shots—or at least a minimum of two shots a day—are the cornerstones of good therapy. For years, based on June's personal experience and that of other diabetics as well as our reading in diabetes literature, we believed that you can't have good control with one shot of NPH a day. But we saw so many diabetics who were on that therapy and who stoutly maintained that they were doing just fine on that one shot and who claimed that their doctors said that was all they needed, that we bit our tongues and said nothing. But recently, at an ADA conference in Wichita, Kansas, we heard one of the nation's most respected diabetologists, Richard Guthrie, speak and he stated flat out that *good control is not possible on one shot of NPH a day.* This is because, as he explained it, while the life of NPH insulin may be twenty-four hours, its therapeutic life (the period during which it controls blood sugar) is only about thirteen hours. With one shot of NPH, therefore, you have eleven hours during which your blood sugar may not be controlled.

This reminded us of the representative of a Danish insulin company who used to squirm at lectures by a well-known diabetologist who is, himself, diabetic. The doctor would point sternly at the rep and say it's all your company's fault that there have been so many diabetics with complications like blindness and kidney failure and amputation. His company's founder had been the one who, years ago, first developed NPH. At that time everyone hailed NPH as a great breakthrough because it meant that rather than taking one shot of regular before each meal, diabetics could take one shot of NPH in the morning and forget about it for the rest of the day. Since blood sugar monitoring was not possible in those days, the one-shot-of-insulin people didn't realize they were running around with high blood sugar a good part (make that a bad part) of the time. The lecturing doctor maintained that many of these people could have avoided the complications they later developed—had they been taking insulin the old-fashioned way with a shot of Regular before each meal.

Now there are many effective insulin therapies using combinations of Regular and NPH or Regular and Lente or Regular and Ultralente. Your doctor can work out the best kind of therapy for you based on how your body works and the kind of life you lead.

In his talk, Dr. Guthrie provided the dismal statistic that up to 80 percent of insulin-taking diabetics are still on one shot of NPH a day. Don't you be one of them.

ADVICE FOR YOU II

Dr. Guthrie also had some wise words of caution for Type II (non–insulin-taking) diabetics. Type IIs have a tendency to think of themselves as having "mild" or "borderline" diabetes, because they don't have to take insulin. This is not true. Type II diabetics may have a different kind of diabetes, a kind that doesn't require insulin, but they are just as diabetic as a Type I. For that reason Type IIs have to take their diabetes as seriously and take just as good care of themselves as their insulin-taking brethren and sistren. This includes taking frequent blood sugar tests. Another time in which we've had to bite our tongues is when a diabetic announces, "My doctor says I only need to test my blood sugar once or twice a week." We'd also heard that, for Type IIs, it's only important to take a fasting blood sugar every morning and if that's in the normal range, that indicates that their control has been good for the last twenty-four hours. After a few weeks of normal blood sugars, the myth continued, then it's okay to drop back to one or two fasting blood sugars a week. Dr. Guthrie laid that myth to rest right beside the one-shot-of-NPH legend. Type IIs blood sugars fluctuate during the course of the day just as much as Type Is and unless the Type IIs take frequent blood sugars (fasting, before and after meals) and provide their doctors with data on their fluctuations, the doctor cannot prescribe the correct dosages of oral hypoglycemic pills and/or make the dietary adjustments necessary for the good control that keeps complications away. Yes, Type II diabetics *can* develop complications just like Type Is if they don't keep their blood sugars in the normal range. The vascular damage can begin when blood sugars are consistently over 150 mg/dl and as Dr. Guthrie points out, this is just as true for both Type I and Type II diabetics.

A_1C A-OK

Another test that all diabetics—whether Type I or Type II—should take regularly is the Hemoglobin A_1C, also known as the glycosylated hemoglobin test. This shows how your overall control has been over approximately the past two to three months by analyzing how much glucose has bonded with the red blood cells. This test is usually performed in the doctor's office. Since the normal range varies with different laboratory tests, rather than asking what the numerical result of your test is, you should ascertain the normal range for that particular laboratory and see where your test fits on the scale.

Recently a home A_1C test has become available. It is called Self-Assure and is made by Evalulab. It's as easy to perform as a standard home blood sugar test, but you send the test to Evalulab for evaluation. Because we wanted to get an idea of the accuracy of a Self-Assure A_1C test, we had June do one and on the same day take one at her doctor's. The results of the tests were virtually identical. Both showed her to be in the normal (nondiabetic) range. On the Self-Assure scale the normal range is 5.9–7.5% and June was 6.8!

We also did another test on Self-Assure to make sure it would get the same results using the same blood. We had Carla, our diabetic nurse-educator, send in two tests made one right after the other. One she sent in with her own name and the other under another name and address. When the test results came back, they were only a tenth of a percent apart!

When we told Evalulab about our successful experiment, they said they remembered June's test because they had run it through twice to make sure nothing was wrong. She said that normal results are so rare among diabetics that they always double-check them!

Naturally, if you should do a Self-Assure test at home, you would want to take it to your doctor for evaluation and to make any necessary changes in your diabetes regimen.

Combining your blood sugar self-testing with regular hemoglobin A_1C tests, you get the total picture of your diabetes—both short-range and long-range. In this way you'll know exactly where you are in terms of control so you'll know where you need to go to in order to be in that select company of diabetics who dwell in the normal range forever.

A-VOIDING URINE TESTS

We've spent most of our time here telling what you ought to do for good control. Now we'll mention something you *can* and *should* give up—urine testing. Since the diabetics we come in contact with are mostly highly motivated people who like to stay on the cutting edge of the latest diabetes therapies, we'd begun to think that nobody does urine testing anymore. But lately we've discovered in our reading and in conversations with diabetes educators that there are still a bunch of urine testers out there in Diabetesland, probably even more than there are people trying to control their diabetes on one shot of NPH a day. Consequently, we'll proceed to lobby for a change.

Urine testing is nonesthetic. Nobody wants to be fooling around with their urine all the time. Children and teenagers especially detest it, much preferring blood sugar testing since that's something you can talk about and even do in public without embarrassment. Friends often ask you to test their blood sugar. Seldom do they request a urine test.

But the negative esthetics of urine testing fade into relative unimportance in comparison to the negative accuracy. As British physician Dr. Tattersall says, "As a means of self-monitoring, urine tests have always been unsatisfactory." In the first place, what you get with a urine test is history. It may show you as having a 195 blood sugar when in reality that's what you had an hour ago, and right now you may be plunging into hypoglycemia. And what if the tape or pill or stick shows you're not spilling? Does that mean your blood sugar is normal or a little above or are you at 50 and falling and about to "go goofy"?

Then there's the formidable problem of the renal threshold, the point at which the kidneys start spilling sugar into the urine. Normally, sugar spills between 150 and 180 but it can vary dramatically from person to person and even from time to time in the same person. For example, older people may find their urine tests are negative when their blood sugar is quite high. June only starts spilling at 220, a fact she didn't discover until she started monitoring her own blood sugar. Younger diabetics may have just the opposite problem. Their renal thresholds are lower and they may be spilling when their blood sugar is normal. Figure 1 shows how the renal threshold changes with age.

As if these weren't accuracy problems enough, there are other ways of getting a false reading from urine tests. Vitamin C and aspirin can both make the test show sugar falsely. Moisture makes test materials deteriorate and give false readings. Even having something sweet on your fingers when you handle the testing materials can affect the test. Clinitest registers other sugars besides glucose. Because of all these factors, you may get a false positive reading when you have no glucose in the urine. And on and on it goes.

FIGURE 1

How "Renal Threshold" Varies with Age*

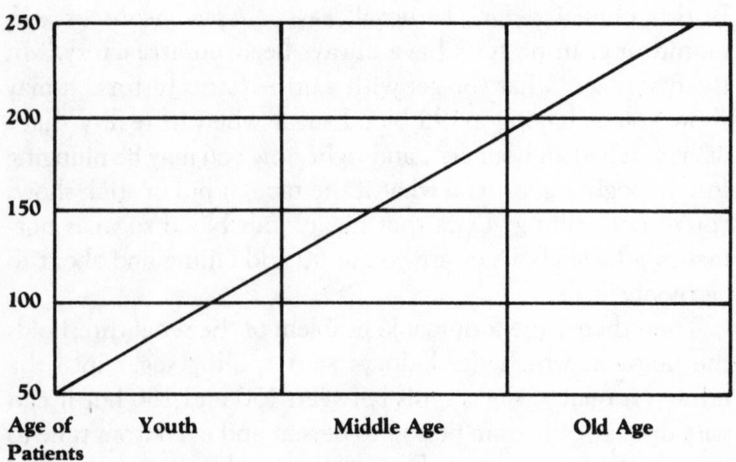

*Courtesy of Charles Weller, M.D., *Diabetes Forecast*, July/August 1978, p. 20.

There's long been the theory that taking a second void is the way to bring more accuracy to urine testing. What you're supposed to do is empty your bladder in the good old-fashioned way, drink a glass of water, and then make your urine test from a sample taken fifteen to thirty minutes later. Although this is a bother, it's supposed to tell you what your blood sugar is at the time of the test.

But "supposed to" ain't necessarily so, as reported in *Diabetes Care.* From the University of Kansas School of Medicine in Wichita, Diana W. Guthrie, Debbie Hinnen, and Richard A. Guthrie deliver the word that shows the ineffectiveness of this extra inconvenience. They discovered that the measurement between the first and second void is seldom significantly different enough to make it worth the trouble. They also point out that the first void actually gives you a better idea of your overall control because it shows if you've been spilling over the last few hours. The second void, taken just before a meal, as is often advised, gives you the lowest-point reading and may falsely lead you to believe you have normal blood sugar even though you may have been spilling heartily two hours earlier.

We know how this works, because back when June did urine testing, when she found herself spilling before a meal, Barbara always suggested that she drink a glass of water and try again to see if she could work down the sugar to an acceptable level so she could eat a normal meal. Then, too, merely drinking a lot of water can affect your reading, because if you have more urine the percentage of sugar will show up as less, even though your blood sugar is the same.

Teenage diabetics figured this one out early on. We heard Los Angeles diabetologist Dr. Robert Rood, who specializes in adolescent diabetes, say that when some of his patients who knew they hadn't been in good control came into the office and were asked to produce a specimen, they'd add a lot of water to it to reduce the percentage of sugar. After they gave the specimen to Dr. Rood, he'd shake hands with them and say, "Congratulations—you're dead." When they looked blank, he'd continue, "Anyone whose urine is as cold as this has to have been dead for twelve hours."

We used to think that urine testing was at least better than no testing at all, but we're changing our minds. When we heard Dr. Jay Skylar, one of the nation's leading diabetologists, speak at an American Association of Diabetes Educators' Conference, he delivered the opinion that urine testing is so inaccurate that he wished that the FDA would withdraw approval of it, since it can be hazardous to your health. We're inclined to agree.

To be fair, though, there are two positives to urine testing. When you are ill or when your blood sugars are running over 250, you should test your urine for ketones. This means your body is converting its fat for fuel, releasing fatty acids which go into the liver where they're converted to ketones. Ketones mean you're dangerously out of control and you should contact your doctor.

David Goldstein, M.D., the eminent diabetologist who developed the Self-Assure test, also told us that a urine test could reveal the fact that you have had some high blood sugar during the course of a period when, according to your blood sugar tests, you appeared to have normal or low blood sugar. Let's say you took your blood sugar at 9:00 A.M. and it was 55, so you took some corrective measures and then didn't test again until just before a noon lunch. That test could be around 100 so your assumption would be that your blood sugar had been low or normal all morning. A urine test that showed sugar would reveal the fact that your blood sugar had gone up high in mid-morning.

Urine tests, then, are useful for ketones and for a super fine-tuning of your control, but they shouldn't be used for your basic testing and certainly shouldn't be used because you're reluctant to stick your finger for the blood sample. A finger-prick is a very minor inconvenience compared to the complications that could develop if you consistently test inaccurately with urine tests. There are many excellent and virtually painless finger-sticking devices on the market now. This makes blood sugar testing a joy compared with back when June first started and had to jab herself with a recycled insulin needle to get the blood sample. If you have trouble getting the blood out of your fingertips, ask your doctor or nurse educator to check your technique. So stick yourself today so you don't get stuck with complications tomorrow. And read on: it may not be too long before you can take your blood sugar without sticking your finger.

Things to Come

As we said previously, new equipment, products, and therapies to aid you in better diabetes control are continually appearing on the scene. It's important for you to keep up on things so that as these new products and therapies arrive, you can jump on them right away to improve your control.

You can read all about these in diabetes publications and the newspapers, but that's not where you find the *very* latest information. The really hot news is in reports you get from stockbrokers concerning new product developments in companies, developments that may cause a stock to go up. We have a few friends in stock brokerages that keep us up-to-date. Thanks to their reports, we heard about the nasal spray insulin before it was common knowledge, the development of a technique for transplanting fetal islet cells, and, most recently, encouraging research on a noninvasive blood sugar test, the infrared beam. (That means you don't have to stick your finger for a drop of blood to take a test.)

It's nice to hear early reports on breakthroughs in diabetes, because it gives you realistic hope that things will be better. But you shouldn't give up the available good therapies and sit around waiting for the newer and better. Most of these will take years before all the problems are worked out and they get FDA approval and will be readily available. Some therapies and instruments, unfortunately, will never make it.

So, for example, don't wait to start testing your blood sugar until you can do it without sticking your finger. By the time that's possible you could have done irreparable damage. Don't even hold off purchasing a meter because you're waiting for the possibly better, possibly smaller, possibly cheaper one that may be just around the corner. That would be akin to never getting a car because next year's model might be improved or less expensive. No, it would be worse than that, because not having a car wouldn't be a threat to your health and well-being. It might even be healthier *not* to have a car because you'd be forced to walk more. Anyway, when it comes to meters, there are almost always advantageous trade-in possibilities for your old meter when new ones come on the scene, so you can usually be assured of being able to upgrade at very little cost.

The thing you should most especially not wait for is a cure. We all know it's coming and it may not be too far away. But don't ignore your diabetes by figuring that it will be cured before too long. A cure will do you very little good if you've neglected your diabetes therapy and developed complications. Take care of your diabetes and take care of your health so you'll be in good shape for the cure and, more important, all the while be in good shape for life!

CHAPTER 2
Diet: Theme and Variations

DIET AS HEALER, DIET AS SLAYER

Kenneth Pelletier, professor of psychology at the University of California, Berkeley, and author of *Mind as Healer, Mind as Slayer,* considers improving the diet to be one of the basic ways of breaking a chronic stress pattern. For a diabetic, diet is even more significant, because besides being a stress maker (or breaker) and health enhancer (or detractor), diet is also an essential component of diabetes therapy. Since diet is, therefore, of such primary importance for a diabetic, we'll put it in the primary position in your building plans for a strong body.

KNOWING BETTER, DOING WORSE

You might call the last ten years the Great American Decade of Dietary Data. Never has so much been written about healthy eating. Newspapers, magazines, and television bombard you with it. Never has a population been made so aware of the need to decrease fat, decrease salt, decrease calories, and increase fish and fiber and fresh fruits and vegetables. Seldom has such good advice been so universally ignored. Marian Burros, food writer for *The New York Times,* in reporting on a 1987 survey of what Americans actually eat, said that most Americans have not "responded in significant fashion . . . to calls for eating more healthfully."

The survey revealed that junk food snacks are still a way of life for most of our citizens and that when push comes to shove it in their mouths, they still take french fries rather than baked potatoes, red meat instead of chicken or fish, and in general choose the nutritionally inferior over the superior.

Food manufacturers may be partially to blame. We notice a strange phenomenon when we attend Fancy Food and Confection Shows and Health Food Expositions seeking out Gourmet Health Foods (foods that are nutritionally healthy and appropriate for diabetics *and* absolutely delicious). While it's true that we do find more foods than ever that meet our stringent requirements, we also notice that practically every food on display is advertised in large letters as being *ALL NATURAL.* A close inspction of the labels reveals that they are often full of all natural sugar, all natural salt, and all natural animal fat as well as all kinds of natural refined ingredients. Misguided souls could erroneously believe that when they eat the "all natural" potato chips fried in coconut oil and the "all natural" chocolate-covered graham crackers that they're doing their bodies a favor.

Another trend is that soft drink manufacturers are starting to advertise that a cola drink is nifty for breakfast. Not that such dietary aberrations really need advertising. People are perfectly capable of figuring them out for themselves. Several months before the cola-for-breakfast campaign was launched, we were in New York for a week, and before doing our morning constitutional in Central Park, we always had our daily breakfast of Irish oatmeal at Rumplemeyer's. The first morning we were there a woman in her early twenties came in for breakfast. Her menu consisted of a cola drink, a cup of coffee with *lots* of sugar, and a milk shake. We thought this was an odd selection but figured she was just indulging in a one-time unnatural craving. But we soon discovered that every day she ordered the identical breakfast. In fact, the counterman always served it to her automatically, just as, after the second day, he always served us our oatmeal without our placing the order.

As a person with diabetes, you can't allow yourself the luxury (*aka* stupidity) of making unhealthy food choices the way the majority of our citizenry are doing. You *have to* make your diet a healer rather than a slayer. It isn't that much of a restriction. Heathly foods can be delicious and, among the growing flowing cornucopia of delicious healthy foods, you can make your selections based on your ethnic traditions and individual taste and even your lifestyle.

MY WAY

When we once went to the Hawaiian Islands on a group tour for diabetics as consultants for diabetic contingencies, a strange phenomenon occurred. Each diabetic who had previously had intimate contact with only one diabetic—him or herself—was thrown into a fairly close relationship with thirteen other diabetics and had an opportunity to watch carefully other diabetics' eating habits and judge them. We noticed that if a diabetic handled diet in a different way from the norm, the other diabetics would decide that that person must be goofing up or goofing off—*not doing it the right way* or "the way I do it."

Some diet-controlled diabetics were appalled at the way the insulin takers would sometimes be discovered lapping up a dish of macadamia-nut ice cream. When we explained that they *needed* ice cream or some other sweet to raise their blood sugar because it was too low, the diet-controlled people would look skeptical. One even suggested that these people were going out of their way to *get* low blood sugar just so they could eat something they weren't supposed to.

The one teenager on the trip struck terror in everyone's heart because she never seemed to sit down and eat a whole well-balanced meal. Despite our urgings, she would pick at her plate and return most of it to the kitchen. We all eyed her nervously, wondering what was feeding her injected insulin. We clutched rolls of Dextrosols (glucose tablets) in our pockets, ready to pop a few into her mouth should she start turning glassy-eyed on us.

Then there was one diabetic who ate quantities of everything. She often downed sweet Hawaiian carbohydrate concoctions that would have sent the average diabetic shooting off the top of the blood-sugar scale. She wasn't overweight and appeared to be healthy. Still, we all expected to find her passed out cold in a diabetic coma with her breath giving off the fruitiness of a grape press as her bloodstream flowed with acetone, the poisonous acid price of her dietary sins.

Then it came to pass that during one of our diabetes-consultant lecture-discussions we were demonstrating how to do one's own blood sugar testing. (This was back in the bad old days before blood sugar testing equipment and supplies were readily available.) And, lo, those who seemed to be flagrant diet violators were well within the normal blood-sugar range. At last everyone relaxed and decided that even if some diabetics didn't do it the "right" way, their way apparently worked for them.

And the offbeat-seeming ways didn't turn out to be all that peculiar, after all. For example, we later found out that the teenager had learned from experience—several hospitalizations—that she couldn't keep in control on three normal-size meals a day. Consequently, she snacked frequently on cheese, crackers, fruit, and especially her beloved "veggies," as she called her collection of raw vegetables. She was doing what was right for her. And that was how we learned that there's more than one way to feed a diabetic cat to make it sleek and glossy, with blood sugar purring along in the normal range.

An Exchange for the Better

Another bad old days (pre–mid-1970s) aspect of diabetes therapy is now mercifully gone forever. Back then when you were definitely diagnosed as diabetic, the doctor—or more likely one of his office minions—pressed into your icy and trembling hand the official American Diabetes Association

Exchange Lists for Meal Planning, saying, in effect, "You are condemned to this." They were printed on one sheet and made it look as if you could never eat a tortilla or bagel or English muffin or grits or pretzels or popcorn again because these choices weren't listed among the Bread Exchanges.

These lists were revised and expanded in 1976 and again in 1986 until now, instead of one sheet, there is a thirty-two-page booklet of food choices plus important information on foods high in fiber (good) and high in sodium (bad). There is also *Exchange Lists for Weight Management,* as well as three special *Guidelines for Use of the Exchange Lists: For Low-Sodium Meal Planning; For Lowfat Meal Planning;* and *For Low-Sodium, Lowfat Meal Planning.*

The ADA also has two menu-planning booklets (with some recipes) to help you figure out calories and exchanges for twenty-eight days' worth of breakfasts, lunches, and dinners: *Month of Meals* and *Month of Meals 2.* All publications mentioned above are available from the American Diabetes Association, 1970 Chain Bridge Road, McLean, VA 22109-0592; phone 1-800-ADA-DISC, extension 363.

In addition, there is *Exchanges for All Occasions* by Marion J. Franz (available from Chronimed, Box 47945, Minneapolis, MN 55447-9727; phone 1-800-876-9540).

The most recommended and most effective approach, however, is to have an individual consultation with an experienced diabetes dietitian who can individualize your eating plan to cater to your diabetes control, to your body's nutritional needs, and to your personal likes and dislikes. For the truth is, no matter how perfect a diet may be for you, if it's full of foods you dislike and empty of foods you like, it's dollars to doughnuts you won't stick to it.

THREE DIETARY ROADS TO DIABETES CONTROL

Even though diets are now preferably tailored to personal tastes, within that framework there are three general dietary directions in which you can go with which to maintain both good blood sugar control and good health. These three diets, each with its own guidebook, represent divergent opinions among health-care professionals. They are what we'll call ADA Exchanges (ADA), High Carbohydrate Fiber (HCF), and High Protein (HP). Each diet has its proponents and its detractors. Many dietitians will offer you a choice among them, since none of the three is really contraindicated for most individuals. We'll lay them out before you here, giving you some of the pros and cons, so that you can wisely weigh them yourself and collaborate with your dietitian or doctor in arriving at the best possible food plan for yourself.

These dietary options differ in the proportion of carbohydrate, protein, and fat recommended and/or in the type of carbohydrate, protein, and fat. All foods are either carbohydrate, protein, or fat—or combinations of the three. (We once read a diet book that said to lose weight you should especially cut back on carbohydrates, proteins, and fat. Yep, that should do it, all right!)

Over the years the ADA and HCF diets have come closer together until they now have more similarities than differences. Briefly we can characterize the three by their proportion of each food component:

	Carbohydrates	**Proteins**	**Fat**
ADA	55–60%	12–20%	25–30%
HCF	55–60%	20%	20–25%
HP	15%	45%	40%

The ADA Exchange Lists are created by committees from the American Diabetes Association and the American Dietetic Association.

The HCF diet was pioneered and perfected by Dr. James Anderson of Lexington, Kentucky. The leading exponent of the High Protein diet is Dr. Richard K. Bernstein of Mamaroneck, New York. Acquainted with both of these physicians for many years, we keep in touch with them and are supportive of both of their theories, although each champions a totally different dietary cause. We like to think of Dr. Anderson's diet as the revolutionary Left (indeed it was when it originally came on the scene, because carbohydrates, which had long been considered the enemy of diabetics, suddenly became the friend). Dr. Bernstein's diet is the radical Right since in the past it used to be that health-conscious people emphasized protein in their diets. The ADA diet is the middle-of-the-road, mainstream plan, the plan most diabetics are introduced to and the plan supported by the large majority of doctors, diabetes educators, and dietitians. Since the ADA Exchange Lists are completely explained in diabetes education classes and are clearly presented in their 1986 booklet we won't re-explain them here; rather we will compare and contrast the lesser-known HCF and HP variations.

The Revolutionary-Left Plan: HCF Diets

The high-carbohydrate, high-fiber diet (HCF) is actually the most ancient of diets for diabetes therapy. More than two thousand years ago a diet rich in legumes (beans, split peas, lentils, etc.) was a common treatment regime for diabetics in India. In the 1950s an Indian doctor, Inder Singh, put a group of his patients on a high-carbohydrate diet and reported that the majority of them lost all symptoms of the disease and that those on insulin quit taking it after three to eighteen weeks. The Japanese have used high-carbohydrate diets (white rice, mainly) as standard treatment for diabetes since the early 1960s.

In this country, Dr. James Anderson of the Veterans' Administration Hospital in Lexington, Kentucky, published in 1984 several studies showing the value of high-carbohydrate, high-fiber diets for his hospital patients. The diet he used with his hospitalized diabetic patients provided 70 percent of calories as carbohydrate, 21 percent as protein, and 9 percent as fat. On these diets insulin doses decreased 38 percent for Type I diabetics and 58 percent for Type II diabetics. (He also found that these diets leveled out blood sugars of people with hypoglycemia.) Reductions in serum cholesterol values were 30 percent for Type I and 24 percent for Type II diabetics. Triglycerides declined 5 percent for Type I and 4 percent for Type IIs.

Dr. Anderson then created a maintenance diet for use outside the hospital, which is what we now know as the HCF diet. He created his own exchanges, which are now available in his booklet, *HCF Exchanges, A Sensible Plan for Healthy Eating.* His exchanges include Starches (grains/vegetables like corn, peas, squash), Garden Vegetables, Fruits, Cereals, Beans, Milk, Proteins, Fats, and Free Vegetables. These exchanges are to be used in conjunction with his manual, *The HCF Guide Book* (Lexington, Kentucky, HCF Diabetes Foundation, 1987).

When Dr. Anderson says carbohydrate, he means *complex* carbohydrate or starches and very few simple sugars—only those in fruits, vegetables, and milk. And when he says fiber, he means carbohydrates packaged in their natural fibrous coating—brown rice instead of white; whole-wheat, rye, or graham flour instead of white; whole cereals like oats, bran, and cracked and shredded wheat; corn, peas, potatoes, beans, and lentils; vegetables like artichokes, bean sprouts, beets, broccoli, eggplant, kale, and squash; and fresh fruit, such as apples, bananas, melons, oranges, peaches, pears, and strawberries rather than fruit juices.

Dr. Anderson's diet gives you 30 to 60 grams of fiber a day (20 to 30 grams per 1,000 calories). Most Americans get only 12 to 20 grams a day. Both the National Academy of Sciences and the FDA now recommend that we should all eat 25 to 30 grams of fiber a day; they also believe that we should eat no more than 35 grams.

Dr. Anderson has compiled a booklet, *Plant Fiber in Foods* (Lexington, Kentucky, HCF Diabetes Foundation, 1986), which gives the fiber content in grams per serving of over 300 common foods. The analyses were made in his own laboratory.

As for protein, the diet allows only a few ounces of the leanest meat, fish, or poultry a day. This is the hardest requirement for most people to follow. Egg yolks are taboo, as are all cheeses except the lowest in fat, like dry cottage, farmer, or hoop cheeses. Fish and poultry (skinned before cooking) are recommended. Meat choices are pretty much limited to lean beef cuts, lean pork, and well-trimmed veal and are to be used more as garnishes and flavorings for vegetables and rice dishes than as main courses.

And now we come to where the dietary belt really gets tightened: the fats. The 1,200-calorie diet has five fat exchanges and only three protein exchanges. You are getting some fat as part of your protein, though Dr. Anderson's exchanges have only two grams of fat, while the American Diabetes Association's (ADA) lean-meat exchanges have three grams. The 2,000-calorie HCF diet allows nine fat exchanges daily (and six protein exchanges). Dr. Anderson recommends cooking with Teflon pans, using Pam (a nonstick vegetable coating for pans), and eliminating oils as much as possible in baking breads and muffins. Milk exchanges are all nonfat.

This brief outline of the way the HCF diet is distinctive from the ADA diet is in no way a picture of what the day's meals are really like. In fact, the big complaint Dr. Anderson gets from his patients the first week is, "I can't eat all that food." And to help you understand why, Table 1 presents a sample day's menus for the 1,800-calorie HCF diet. Besides the foods listed, coffee, tea, and other low-calorie beverages are allowed as desired.

Eyes bulging in disbelief at the amount of carbohydrates, you are probably reacting as June first did: "This is nutritional suicide." But you're mistaken. This diet is simply a different and, for some of you, possibly a better way to handle your health and possibly your diabetes. But before you decide to "HCF it," here are some pros and cons for you to consider.

Table 1. Sample Meal Plan for 1,800-Calorie Maintenance Diet

From J. W. Anderson and Kyleen Ward, "Long-Term Effects of High-Carbohydrate, High-Fiber Diets on Glucose and Lipid Metabolism: A Preliminary Report on Patients with Diabetes," *Diabetes Care*, March/April 1978, p. 79.

Meal	Food Item	Portion Size	Weight (Grams)
Breakfast	Bran buds	⅔ cup	60
	Banana	½	50
	Whole-wheat toast	2 slices	46
	Skim milk	1 cup	240
	Corn-oil margarine	1 tsp.	5
10:00 A.M. snack	Whole-wheat muffin	1	60
Noon meal	White-bean soup	1 cup	200
	Hash-brown potatoes	½ cup	100
	Stewed tomatoes	¾ cup	150
	Pickled beets	½ cup	100
	Fresh apple, cored	1 small	100
	Whole-wheat bread	1 slice	23
	Corn-oil margarine	2 tsp.	10
Evening meal	Roast beef	3 oz.	90
	Baked potato	1 small	100
	Corn	½ cup	75
	Carrots	½ cup	75
	Salad: lettuce	1½ cups	100
	cucumber	1 medium	100
	zero dressing*	1 tbsp.	15

*This specially prepared low-calorie dressing contains four calories per tablespoon.

	Peaches, water-packed	½ cup	100
	Whole-wheat muffin	1	60
	Corn-oil margarine	1 tsp.	5
Evening snack	Whole-wheat muffin	1	60

The Pros

Insulin Elimination or Reduction. We hate to even mention the idea of insulin elimination because some of you will feel that's such a pro it will outweigh any con we can come up with. But we're talking facts and here are the facts, as stated by Dr. Anderson himself.

> For lean diabetic individuals VERY GOOD responses are likely for adults with good glycemic control using diet, oral hypoglycemic agents *or* less than 25 units of insulin daily. With HCF diets most of those taking oral hypoglycemic agents can discontinue them and over one-half of those taking insulin can discontinue it and maintain good glycemic control with diet and exercise. HCF diets lower serum cholesterol by 20% and triglycerides by 10–25%.
>
> GOOD responses are likely for adults with good glycemic control using 25–40 units of insulin daily. . . . Average insulin doses can be decreased about 33% and insulin reactions are less frequent. HCF diets lower average serum cholesterol by 20% and triglycerides by 10–25%.
>
> FAIR responses to HCF diets are observed for lean individuals treated with over 40 units of insulin daily, for

those with a history of diabetic ketoacidoses, or for those individuals with Type I diabetes. Reductions of insulin doses average 10–15%. Insulin reactions tend to be less frequent and glycemic control is somewhat improved. The major benefits relate to the 20% reduction in average serum cholesterol concentrations and the 10–15% reduction in triglycerides.

Please notice that all Type I diabetics fall into the FAIR responses group.

When we come to obese diabetic individuals, here is what Dr. Anderson has to say:

> The major problem for the obese diabetic individual is peripheral resistance to insulin action. Giving exogenous insulin does not correct this problem. The measures that overcome peripheral resistance to insulin or increase insulin sensitivity are: weight reduction, high carbohydrate/fiber diets, exercise, and sulfonylurea agents (pills).
>
> Theoretically, then, the best approach to obesity with diabetes is a high carbohydrate/fiber, weight-reducing diet combined with an exercise program. The sulfonylurea agents may be useful adjuncts for selected individuals. We have used this therapeutic approach for ten years.

In his clinical studies, Dr. Anderson's program resulted in 52 percent of the obese insulin-taking diabetics being taken off insulin completely.

For the most skeptical of you we might add another comment from Dr. Anderson: "These diets have not increased insulin requirements in any patients."

We would also add that it is dangerous to change to this diet without working with your physician. Insulin dosages must be lowered cautiously and *slowly*. When starting individuals on his diet, Dr. Anderson requires that they be in control first; then he lowers the dosage by 10 percent or 2 to 4 units.

Weight-Reduction Benefits. Most of you diabetics—some say as many as 85 percent—are the maturity-onset, non–insulin-dependent variety and a great proportion of you can control your diabetes without using either insulin or pills. All you have to do to stay symptom-free is to lower your weight and keep it down, control your calories, and avoid concentrated sweets. If you're this kind of diabetic, the HCF diet could help you immensely, because it is an effective reducing diet.

Dr. Anderson is careful to make no wild claims for it even in this respect, however, saying conservatively, "Many of our patients are able to lose weight on these HCF diets. The secret to weight loss on these diets is to reduce total calories by cutting out sugar (sucrose) and greatly restricting the intake of all fats and oils."

We have found, however, that the diet works like magic at making pounds disappear. Barbara, who had gradually gained ten pounds over her ideal weight and had unsuccessfully tried several different diet-deprivation techniques to get them off, went on the 1,500-calorie HCF diet when June did and within six weeks the pounds disappeared pleasantly and painlessly, because . . .

You Are Never Hungry. When we talk to diabetes groups, one of the complaints we hear most frequently from Type IIs who are conscientiously following a diet to lose weight is, "I'm always starved." We particularly remember a time when we were explaining the joys of the Exchange Lists and how you can eat almost anything if you just know what's in it and calculate your diet accordingly. One woman raised her hand and said, sadly, "I'm going to Italy and I won't be able to have pasta." "Oh, yes, indeed you can," said June with a cheerful smile. "You can have half a cup of it for your bread exchange."

"That's not enough," was the woman's terse response.

With the HCF diet the woman could have doubled or even tripled that. Of course, she could have had only a teaspoon of oil and no cheese or cream on it . . . but that's a story for the "con" section later.

In essence, though, being on the HCF diet is never having to say you're hungry, and for a diabetic with a weight problem that's a lot not to have to say.

Lower Food Bills. The HCF diet costs about 30 percent less than the normal diet. You get a lot more vegetables, grains, and legumes for your money than you do meat, fish, and cheese. Since a great number of diabetics are in their retirement years on fixed incomes, the lowered cost of food alone is a heavy plus.

A Healthier Diet. You read about it every other day. The American diet is unhealthy, primarily because it's too high in fats (particularly saturated fats) and meats, and too low in complex carbohydrate and fiber. In other words, to be healthy the American diet should become the HCF diet. The low-fat-diet concept is being emphasized for all Americans and especially for diabetics, as is the low-saturated-fat idea, because fat boosts blood cholesterol and triglycerides (blood fats), both of which contribute to the cardiovascular problems to which diabetics are particularly susceptible.

But that's not the end of the fat story for diabetics. It is now thought that in overweight Type II diabetics the problem is not lack of insulin but the inability of insulin to get into the cells, what Dr. Anderson calls "peripheral resistance to insulin." These diabetics often have abnormally *high* insulin levels in their blood. Excessive fat in the blood may well be what prevents the insulin from being used. As Dr. Anderson says, "For many diabetics, the fat in their diet is their worst enemy. Eating fat blocks the action of insulin—the body cannot burn sugar very well after a meal containing a lot of fat."

Another problem with fats is that they make you fat. Fat is two and a quarter times higher in calories than either carbohydrate or protein. Fat has nine calories per gram while carbohydrate and protein have only four.

The coup de grace for fat, as far as we're concerned, is that all the chemical culprits of modern agriculture and pollution tend to be stored in animal fat. That makes a pretty solid case for a low-fat diet.

The high-fiber aspect of the diet is another old idea whose time has come again. Fiber was a basic component of diets of yore when refining and processing weren't in flower—or flour. Fiber is also high in the diets of primitive tribes in such places as Africa. A British physician, Dr. Dennis Burkitt, helped fiber make its comeback by reporting on the low incidence among the African tribespeople of those common American problems of cardiovascular disease, cancer of the colon, diverticulosis, ulcerative colitis, varicose veins, and gall bladder disease. If fiber helps prevent all this, you can see what a total health product it is.

Again we'll give Dr. Anderson the last word on the particular benefits of fiber for diabetics:

> Eating plant fibers . . . improves glucose and fat metabolism. Starches and sugars are more slowly absorbed when they are eaten as part of a high-fiber diet. Thus, the blood sugar does not go as high after a high-fiber meal as it does after low-fiber meals.
>
> Several plant fibers lower blood-cholesterol values in a dramatic fashion. Beans and oatmeal have the type of fibers that lower the blood-cholesterol level. Our HCF diets lower the blood-cholesterol levels by an average of fifty points (50 mg./100 ml.).
>
> High-fiber diets also tend to lower blood triglycerides. Because plant fibers lower the blood fats they may be beneficial in preventing heart disease and hardening of the arteries.

More Vitamins and Minerals. The foods you eat in greatest quantity on the HCF diet are exactly the ones that are the richest in vitamins and minerals. Whole-grain bread, that great repository of B vitamins and trace elements, is another example.

And, of course, the heaps of vegetables deliver even more on the vitamin and mineral line.

The Cons

Highs and Lows. Now, after making it sound as if the HCF plan is possibly the Messiah of diets for all diabetics, we feel we should reveal a few flies in this all-healing ointment. In the first place, the HCF diet takes some physical getting used to. Everybody who goes on it experiences strange stomach rumblings and excessive flatulence (gas) during the adjustment period. This eventually passes—in every sense of the word—but until it does many people find it distressing.

During your adjustment period, as a diabetic you may record a few high blood sugars from the unusual amounts of carbohydrate. This is a transition stage. Later—as your insulin needs start going down—you experience frequent low-blood-sugar incidents. These unpredictable highs and lows and changes are why you have to work so closely with your doctor as you embark upon the HCF diet.

Actually, the ideal way to go on the HCF diet is to spend two weeks in the hospital having your blood sugar monitored by Dr. Anderson and your body fed exactly the right meals by Beverly Sieling, his dietitian. But, since so few of us are veterans who happen to live in Lexington, Kentucky, and can be admitted to the VA hospital there where both of them work, this is not a practical solution.

It's Un-American. Every diabetes book you read (including ours) and every diabetes lecture you attend make a point of insisting that you *can* live a "normal" life as a diabetic. Nevertheless, in our steak and hamburger and hot dog and pizza and ice cream culture, the HCF diet is simply not the "normal" American diet. You particularly realize this when you try to dine in restaurants or eat in fast-food chains. Meat arrives in gross hunks. When you can only eat two or three ounces of it, you wind up with more in your doggie bag than in your stomach. Fat is everywhere—sludging up the salad, drowning the vegetables, blobbed over potatoes, melting onto warm rolls, and invisibly lurking in everything. You have to ask the waiter for so many things on the side that you hardly have anything in the middle.

As for fiber, it's nonexistent. Most restaurant fare is composed of foods that have been processed to a fare-thee-well or, more accurately, fare-thee-ill. Even in health-food and vegetarian restaurants that purport to practice coscientious cookery you can't escape the fat. It's cheese-this and nuts-that and avocado-the-other thing.

And all diabetics already know the obstacle course of trying to keep to their diets while dining at the homes of friends. The HCF plan is possible only if you have diet-conscious friends or are most intimate with vegetarians and those in the know about nutrition.

Meat and cheese, incidentally, are what most people miss the most on the HCF diet. Meat is what too many American meals still revolve around. Cheese is many people's favorite protein, but you're restricted to the relatively fat-free varieties such as low-fat cottage cheese, ricotta, part-skim-milk mozzarella, and all the special low-fat, low-cholesterol cheeses now on the market like *Lifetime.* Happily, many of these new low-fat cheeses are quite delicious and melt well in cooking.

Psychological Deprivation. Since the body and mind are so intimately interrelated, there can be some psychological problems associated with the HCF diet. For those who feel breakfast isn't breakfast without bacon and eggs, for example, then breakfast *isn't* breakfast and they go around feeling unsatisfied all day long. As another example, for diabetic teenagers, who have already given up so much of being dietetically one of the gang, to have to forgo the ubiquitous hamburgers, French fries, and pizza as well can become the lump of coal on top of the deprivation sundae.

No matter how healthy and slenderizing the HCF diet would be for the entire family (and it would be), it won't be easy to get them—without the goad of diabetes—to make the "sacrifices" this diet involves. And it's not easy to prepare the HCF diet for one member of the family and the "normal" diet for everyone else.

In fact, it's not easy to fix the HCF diet for anyone. It involves cooking lots of pots of beans and soups and cutting up vegetables and baking from scratch and shopping daily for fresh fruits and vegetables. Dr. Anderson himself has come to realize that, as he says, "high-fiber diets are not for everyone."

Still, it *can* be done; but if you feel your life is already unbelievably cluttered with thoughts and activities related to diabetes, then no matter how effective and revitalizing and therapeutic the HCF would be for you, it probably *isn't* for you.

The Radical Right: Low-Carbohydrate, High-Protein Diet

The radical-right eating pattern is a method of treatment described in detail in Dr. Richard K. Bernstein's two books, *Diabetes: The GlucoGraf Method for Normalizing Blood Sugar* (1983) and *Diabetes Type II: Living a Long, Healthy Life through Blood Sugar Normalization* (1990). The first book is intended only for Type I diabetics, while the second is directed toward Type IIs, but also includes newer, updated information and techniques for Type Is.

Dr. Bernstein is known among his medical colleagues as the "Tartar of tight control." He is dead set against a high-carbohydrate diet because carbohydrates raise blood sugar as well as cholesterol and triglycerides in diabetics. His latest book cites studies in the late '80s that "demonstrated lower levels of blood glucose and improved blood lipids [fats] when patients were put on lower-carbohydrate, high-fat diets." His contention is that "the evidence is now overwhelming that elevated blood glucose is a major cause of high serum lipid levels and, more significantly, the major factor in high rates of various heart diseases associated with diabetes."

Dr. Bernstein has never been reluctant to go against the current. We'd even say he positively enjoys the role of iconoclast and because he does, he has been responsible for several innovative breakthroughs in diabetes therapy. Diabetic himself since the age of twelve, he was always on the alert for ways to improve his therapy. In 1971 he discovered the existence of a blood glucose monitor (Ames Eyetone). Since it was a prescription item, he had his psychiatrist wife purchase one for him and he began testing his own blood sugar on a daily basis. With the meter he devised a new self-management method which involved six blood sugar tests a day and doses of Regular (fast-acting) insulin before each meal, along with some Ultralente (long-range) insulin for long-range control instead of the conventional one shot of NPH a day.

Using his own method, he was able to keep his blood sugar within the normal range 90 percent of the time. He also discovered that protein did not raise his blood sugar after meals as fast or as much as carbohydrate, and this, too, he incorporated into his program.

Since he soon realized that in order for his discoveries to make an impact on the diabetes therapy scene he'd have to have the right credentials, at the age of forty-five he resigned his corporate executive position and enrolled in the Albert Einstein College of Medicine and there earned his medical degree.

Now, at fifty-six and after forty-four years of living with diabetes, Dr. Bernstein has no diabetes complications, except a minor foot deformity and some hardening of the arteries left over from the days before he devised his own therapy. We got acquainted with him in 1976 as one of the 150 collaborators on our *Diabetic's Sports and Exercise Book.* At that time he introduced June to blood sugar self-testing, and she gives him credit for the fact that after twenty-five years of diabetes she has not had a single complication.

Dr. Bernstein's rationale for his diet is that carbohydrates must be kept at a minimum because they cause rapid rises in blood sugar. Protein, on the other hand, is converted much more slowly to glucose and does not cause rapid rises in blood sugar. He feels that fat is safe because it has no effect on blood sugar. The chart in Appendix A, reprinted from his book, shows how long it takes different types of carbohydrate and protein to be converted to glucose during metabolism and how long it takes the glucose to disappear from the blood.

Dr. Bernstein and the patients he has trained are able to keep their blood sugars absolutely normal after eating. He does not even approve of rises of up to 150 after a meal, as many endocrinologists do. These are his guidelines for a diet that slows the rise in blood sugar after a meal:

1. Total elimination of foods that contain simple sugars.
2. Limitation of total carbohydrate intake to an amount that will not cause a postprandial (after eating) blood glucose rise or, in Type IIs, overwork the already depleted reserve of pancreatic cells that produce insulin (beta cells).
3. Stopping eating before you feel stuffed (though there is no need to leave the table feeling hungry).

The typical carbohydrate distribution for the day's meals (examples appear in parentheses) is:

Breakfast: 6 grams of carbohydrate (¼ bagel)
Lunch: 12 grams of carbohydrate (2 cups of salad)
Dinner: 12 grams of carbohydrate (⅓ cup pasta)

Protein is whatever amount you like (for example: breakfast—2 oz., lunch—4 oz., dinner—6 oz.), but the amounts per meal must be consistent every day. The amount of fat can vary from meal to meal, but watch total calories if you are overweight.

As Dr. Bernstein points out, keeping track of grams of carbohydrate and ounces of protein requires far less effort than following the Exchange System. And, in fact, counting carbohydrates is a system now recommended for people on the insulin infusion pump and a system that June worked out for herself years ago.

Finally, let us give you a picture of what you don't eat on Dr. Bernstein's diet—allowing, of course, for individual variations. Here is his list of foods to avoid: powdered sweeteners; most so-called diet food and sugar-free food (except diet sodas, sugar-free Jell-O-brand gelatin desserts, and No-Cal-brand syrups); fruits and fruit juices (including tomato and vegetable juices); desserts and pastries; milk, cream, and cottage cheese; powdered milk substitutes and coffee lighteners; snack foods (pretzels, potato chips, crackers, and so forth); candies, including sugar-free brands; cold cereals, except ½ cup puffed wheat; hot cereals; most commercially prepared soups; cooked carrots, cooked potatoes, cooked corn, beets; bread, crackers, and other flour products (some diabetics can tolerate small amounts); pancakes and waffles; cooked tomatoes, tomato paste, and tomato sauce; honey and fructose; most so-called health foods; white and brown rice; pasta and wild rice (though these may be consumed in small amounts).

So what do you eat? You eat vegetables; meat, fish, fowl, and eggs; cheeses; soy milk; nuts; zero-carbohydrate soups; yogurt, soybean flour; soybean bacon, sausages, hamburger, and steak; GG Scandinavian bran crispbread and Bran-a-Crisp; coffee, tea, seltzer, mineral water, club soda, diet sodas; mustard, pepper, salt, spices, herbs; table sweeteners like saccharin, aspartame, and cyclamates; zero-carbohydrate chewing gum; toasted *nori*; frozen diet-soda pops; very low carbohydrate desserts (recipes appear in his book); alcohol in very limited amounts and of very limited kinds.

When it comes to fats, Dr. Bernstein wants his patients to minimize them, especially saturated fats. But he believes that "loading with carbohydrate will probably be more harmful in the long run than loading with fats."

As for fiber, he again goes against the mainstream. To him fiber consumption is of no special benefit to diabetics. He claims that the haphazard use of food high in fiber can be harmful to blood sugar control in Type I diabetics. He acknowledges the fact that plant fiber does appear to reduce postprandial blood sugar elevation in some diabetics who still produce part of their own insulin and in some Type IIs, but that's as far as he will go in joining the high-fiber school of thought.

Dr. Bernstein is not alone in this view. Though Dr. Anderson and others have shown the many health benefits of fiber, its lowering effect on blood sugar is still debatable. Marion Franz, R.D., in "Your Fiber Guide: Understanding What Fiber Is and How It Helps," published in *Diabetes Forecast* (January 1988), wrote, "Nor is it clear . . . how reliable a tool fiber can be for helping to control blood-sugar levels in people with diabetes." Once again, the only way to see if fiber helps or hinders you is to make your own tests with high-fiber foods. For example, compare your blood sugar after a measured serving of beans with what it is after your usual carbohydrate serving at lunch, and see what happens. That's the acid test.

A final consideration about the High Protein diet is its effect on the kidneys. Even high-performance athletes are being warned that increasing protein does not increase their strength or promote muscle building. Increased protein, evidence shows, has no relationship to fitness. They are also cautioned that too much protein and/or taking amino acid supplements can be harmful. It can cause long-term damage to kidneys and interfere with normal digestion of protein. Most Americans already consume twice as much protein as they need. The recommended dietary allowance (RDA) of protein for an adult is eight-tenths of a gram for each kilogram of body weight. A man weighing 180 pounds (82 kilograms) needs about 65 grams of protein a day. In an example Dr. Bernstein gives in his first manual, a patient eating a 1,500-calorie-per-day diet would eat 57 grams of protein in one 499-calorie meal.

Physical Benefits. The obvious and greatest benefit of Dr. Bernstein's diet and method of handling diabetes is that blood sugar is normal (80 to 90 mg./dl) an overwhelming percentage of the time. This means the elimination of what he calls "the tragedy of diabetes"—such complications as blindness, kidney failure, and foot or leg amputation from gangrene. The release from fear of these so-called inevitables can't help but alleviate a formidable stress of the ongoing, unrelieved, most destructive kind for those children and adults who have tried in vain to control their blood sugars and have heretofore found no solution to their problem.

An Imprudent Diet. For born-again diet freaks like us, the diet of the program with its high protein and fat and low carbohydrate and fiber seems downright unhealthy. Indeed, in certain respects it's the direct opposite of the recommendations of the American Diabetes Association, the American Heart Association, the American Cancer Association, and the National Research Council.

The High Protein diet is particularly inadvisable for those who already have kidney damage. Cookbooks for diabetics on dialysis all feature low-protein diets (below 50 grams a day) because protein makes the kidneys work harder. Kidney function also declines with age, and this means that older people should, if anything, lower the amount of protein they eat.

And one more caveat: excess protein can cause you to lose calcium and therefore promote bone loss, particularly inadvisable to post-menopausal women who are already at risk for osteoporosis.

Although we don't follow the High Protein diet ourselves, we know that some diabetics may well have good reason to march to the beat of this different drummer.

Indexing Your Carbohydrates

In 1983, the Glycemic Index hit the news. Based on research by Dr. David Jenkins of the University of Toronto, this is a gauge of how fast and far certain foods raise your blood sugar. The Glycemic Index is by no means a diet like the ADA or HCF or High Protein. First, it lists only sixty-two foods, and many of these (e.g., Mars candy bars) are hardly diabetic dietary staples. Second, as Dr. Jenkins himself pointed out, there are other things to consider in selecting foods besides how they raise—or don't raise—your blood sugar.

Still, the Glycemic Index is something every diabetic should be aware of since it gives you guidelines in food selection and reveals some surprising facts: carrots, for example, raise your blood sugar twice as fast as orange juice, and yams and sweet potatoes have much less effect on your blood sugar than white potatoes.

Everyone who likes to use the Glycemic Index as a guide is waiting eagerly for more foods to be analyzed and listed (although their eagerness may be cooling down a little since no new foods have been analyzed and listed since the initial introduction of the index).

Phyllis Crapo, R.D., the dietitian who has done more than anyone else in America to elucidate the Glycemic Index, believes that since everyone's body reacts in slightly different ways to different foods, what we should do is create our own Glycemic Index by eating various foods and testing our blood sugar afterward. This way you can find out which specific foods tend to raise your blood sugar most so you can avoid them. See Appendix B for a copy of the Glycemic Index.

AFTER THE REVOLUTION

The German philosopher Hegel theorized that changes in thought and history take place through the dialectic process. You start with a thesis—the way things are. Then you add antithesis—the changes advocated by revolutionaries. And finally you arrive at synthesis—the combining of the best or at least the most workable parts of both. This synthesis then becomes the new thesis for future revolutionaries to work on.

Changes in diabetes management happen in somewhat the same way. In order to help you work out your own new diabetes total-health dialectic, it may help to show how June has synthesized the two revolutionary methods with her previous, more conventional program and worked out her own current synthesis.

June's diet is somewhat left of the ADA Exchange List Diet Center, but not quite as far left as the HCF. If she had more time available to cook beans and grains and prepare new and exciting vegetable dishes, she would undoubtedly go farther and farther left, since that's her basic dietary inclination. As far as fat in the diet is concerned, she's almost total HCF. We have a friend who was on a weight-loss program, one aspect of which was fat-aversion therapy. They showed movies of such things as fat-oozing bacon with a commentary about how nasty and disgusting all this greasy stuff is. At the end of the program, the participants were supposed to react with horror and flee from any fat that appeared on their plates. If there is such a thing as reincarnation, then June must have attended several of these fat-aversion therapy sessions in previous lives because there is no one who is as repelled by fat as she. She drinks only nonfat milk, puts no butter or butter substitute on her bread, detests fried food of all kinds, can't stand barbecued ribs, and practically puts on salad dressing with an eyedropper. This is probably why she has never in her life had a weight problem, and also why, when she loses weight because of minor illnesses like the flu, she has a great deal of trouble putting it back on.

June has also synthesized the multiple injections of the Bernstein method into her therapy. From almost as soon as she heard about it, she got onto the combination of Regular and Ultralente before breakfast, Regular before lunch, and Regular and Ultralente before dinner, with occasional extra small injections of Regular on the rare occasions when her blood sugar is temporarily out of control. This has worked beautifully as far as control is concerned and magnificently as far as flexibility of lifestyle, since she no longer has to eat on a rigid time schedule.

When formulating your own synthesis from the dietary antitheses, there is one thing to remember. It may be obvious, but we'll say it anyway: you can't have the HCF diet one meal and Bernstein's high-fat-and-protein diet the next. You have to make a commitment. You can't say, "For lunch I'll have a big bowl of bean soup and some bread and corn on the cob, but for supper I'll change plans and have a steak and a salad with a lot of blue cheese dressing." The HCF diet won't work if you alternate it with meals containing all that fat and protein, and the Bernstein plan won't work with all that carbohydrate. Your poor body won't know what to do and your poor diabetes will be swinging in all directions.

Therefore, if you can't totally commit yourself to one or the other, it's best to stay with the standard Exchange Lists; they represent a synthesis of the two extremes, but it is a balanced synthesis in each meal and therefore keeps your body and your diabetes on an even keel.

CHAPTER 3
Diet: Cautionary Notes

No matter which diet plan or combination of plans you elect to follow, there are certain basic principles of dietary health that apply to all diabetics. In fact, most of these apply in large measure to all nondiabetics as well. Therefore, if you can convince your family members and friends to join you in your general dietary-improvement plan, you'll be giving them a tremendous gift of well-being. You'll also be helping yourself because it's a lot less difficult to make changes for the better in your diet if those around you aren't chomping on the health underminers we all know and love.

THREE FOR THE ROAD TO OBLIVION

In western movies you can always tell the good guys because they wear the white hats. In your diet, it doesn't work that way. Three of the worst culprits who are out to gun down your health are white as the driven snow—sugar, salt, and white flour.

Bitter Sweets

It should give you some measure of comfort to know that even if you weren't a diabetic you should shun sugar as much as you have to because you are. In fact, sugar is so bad for everyone that we've heard it said if sugar were just discovered today the FDA would have to ban it because of its many detrimental effects on health.

If you want to turn yourself off sugar so completely that you shriek in terror when you pass a sugar display in the supermarket and recoil from a candy bar as if from a viper, read *Sugar Blues* by William Dufty. He blames that "simple" $C_{12}H_{22}O_{11}$—the simple sugar called sucrose—for every woe and evil of humankind, including acne, menstrual cramps, cancer, depression, alcoholism, ulcers, schizophrenia, and the decline and fall of all the major civilizations in the history of the world.

Dufty, of course, is a fanatic, but even nonfanatics agree that sugar makes you fat, sugar gives you cavities, sugar rasies your blood pressure, sugar increases your chances of blood-clotting problems in the veins, sugar depletes your B vitamins, and sugar ups your triglycerides. On top of all that, sugar is addictive (worse than opium and its derivatives, opines Dufty). It has been called by some the "alcoholism of children."

One secret of business success is to "find something you can make for a nickel, sell for a dollar, and is habit-forming." A lot of manufacturers of sweet products have discovered this secret. They are flailing us with advertising about their sugar-shot merchandise, and they're putting sugar in almost everything these days. That's why it's so tough to avoid sugar in our society. Sugar is such an accepted, even approved, additive in foods that it's actually illegal to label a product ketchup if it doesn't contain sugar. (Trader Joe's, a food-store chain in Southern California, markets its own brand of "ketchup," which is sugar-free. They have to call it "Ketchy" to get around the law.) Apparently the ketchup producers aren't required to call sugar by name, however. On one label we saw it euphemized to "natural sweetener."

As a diabetic you have the advantage of not being able to consume the quantities of sugar that most people thoughtlessly load up on. These quantities average out to 500 calories of sugar per person *every day*. Teenagers top even that. They consume almost 10,500 calories (close to three pounds!) of sugar a week. For diabetics the American Diabetes Association now approves of up to one teaspoon of sugar per reasonable serving of food. The maximum number of teaspoons per day depends on personal calorie allotment. This sugar is allowable only combined with food, and only if your blood sugar is in control.

The Sweet Alternatives. Many diabetics turn their lives into an unending quest for sweets that don't count—sweets that don't cause damage either diabetically or otherwise. As a homely philosopher has said, "There's no such thing as a free lunch"—and there's no such thing as a free sweetener.

First the cyclamates came under suspicion and finally appeared on the forbidden list. We're not going to debate here whether cyclamates will or will not cause cancer in humans just because huge amounts do so in laboratory mice. But no matter whether cyclamates deserve their ban, they're gone until the manufacturer gets reapproval, which it is seeking.

Saccharine has been under the gun since 1977, but Congress keeps delaying its ban. The U.S. Senate passed another five-year moratorium on its ban in 1987.

The more recent entries into the so-called noncaloric-sweetener field (actually they do have a few calories, about four per table packet) are aspartame, which we're all familiar with as NutraSweet, and acesulfame-K (Ace-K), with the brand name Sunette, marketed as Sweet One and Swiss Sweet. Aspartame is now used in an almost endless array of commercial products from cereals to soft drinks, and the list keeps expanding with new FDA approvals. Its drawback is that it can't be used in cooking, as it loses its sweetness when heated. It can be added only after cooking. Another problem is that rumblings about its safety keep surfacing, though the Centers for Disease Control has found no connection between reported side effects and aspartame.

Ace-K's advantage is that you can cook with it, although it

does not have the volume or texture of sugar (important in baking).

Other new sugar substitutes on the way are sucralose, alitame, and about five others. The more the merrier, because using a variety means you won't overload on any one and risk physical side effects.

Three substances sometimes touted as ideal sweeteners for diabetics are the so-called nutritive sugar substances: fructose, HSH, and the sugar alcohols sorbitol and mannitol. HSH (hydrogenated starch hydrolysate) is chemically the same as sorbitol. They're called nutritive not because they teem with things that are good for you, but because they contain calories and carbohydrates and therefore cannot be thrown into and onto your food without being counted.

Their advantage over cyclamates, saccharine, and aspartame is that they have not been found to cause cancer in mouse bladders or seizures in people. These sweeteners also have the advantage of acting more like table sugar (sucrose) in cooking and baking. And they don't have a bitter aftertaste.

The advantages of these nutritive sugar substitutes for diabetics are that they are absorbed more slowly, and that in the first stages of metabolization they do not require insulin. Because of this, they don't cause blood sugar to rise as rapidly after eating. (Fructose will raise your blood sugar exactly as sugar does, if your blood sugar is already high!) They also seem to be less inclined to raise cholesterol and triglyceride levels than table sugar is.

A disadvantage of the sugar alcohols is that in anything other than very small amounts they can cause diarrhea—not a happy event for anyone, but especially hazardous for a diabetic. According to the manufacturers of products containing HSH, it does not have as pronounced a laxative effect.

In our opinion, the best of the bunch is fructose. Because it's one and a half times sweeter than sugar and three times sweeter than sorbitol you can use less of it for the same sweetness. Also, it *is* a natural product. In England it's called "fruit sugar" and the British Diabetic Association recommends it as the ideal cooking sweetener for diabetics. In fact, in England and in Europe it really is made from fruit, while in the United States it is made from corn. Although chemically fructose is the same in both varieties, some people claim there is a taste difference. You can purchase fructose in liquid or granular form. It has virtually the same calorie count as sugar, about 110 calories an ounce.

Not to overdo the virtues of fructose, let us point out that although it is considered a fruit exchange it is nevertheless one without the fiber and nutritive advantages of fruit. A tablespoon of fructose does not seem like a good trade for a fresh, juicy peach or ten large, sweet cherries or a small, crunchy apple. Fructose, in short, is not the free lunch you've been looking for.

What is a diabetic to do, then, to satisfy the sweet tooth that some diabetics seem to have? Rather than trying to satisfy it, we think you should just yank the rotten rascal out by the roots. Get yourself to the point where you no longer like excessively sweet things. Change your taste.

It can be done. In her prediabetic days, June was as hooked on her midmorning sweet roll, her Sunday pancakes and syrup as anybody. But gradually over the years her taste for sweet things, except for the natural sweetness of fruit, has left her. It took no tremendous strength of character on her part. It just happened. Now she has about one artificially sweetened soda every six months, if that. She puts fresh fruit and/or cinnamon on cereal, never sugar or artificial sweeteners. When she occasionally wants a little jam for her home-baked oat bran muffins, she uses one of the many preserves or jellies that are made totally of fruit.

If you can keep yourself from being obsessed by your "great loss" of sweets, from constantly regretting the long-gone pie à la mode, you'll probably find it wasn't such a great loss after all. You'll actually begin to discover subtle nuances of flavors that were previously buried by overloads of sugar or artificial sweeteners.

Sweet 'n Low Blow and Equal. Those little pink and blue packets you find on restaurant tables with the sugar are not as innocent as they look. If you take a magnifying glass and read the list of ingredients in either Sweet 'n Low or Equal, you'll find that dextrose (glucose) is the leading ingredient. Does this mean you should avoid them, even though they're supposedly for dieters and diabetics? Our diabetic diabetes dietitian at the SugarFree Center says one or two won't hurt you. The dextrose is there only to provide bulk and there is too little of it to be concerned if you limit yourself to a small amount in your coffee or tea. This makes a question pop into mind. How then can these be called sugar substitutes, considering what they contain?

This product and others can be designated as sugar-free or sugar substitute because in the United States the food-labeling laws identify sugar as sucrose. Glucose, fructose, maltose, ribose, mannose, etc. are not legally sugar.

You can see from this how many "sugar-free" products are loaded with things that are sugar for all intents and purposes, except legal ones. You have to be very astute in your label reading: keep an eye out for names like xylose, mannose, dextrose, glucose, sucrose, fructose, sorbitol, mannitol, xylitol, etc. And while you're at it, keep an eye out for honey. It's as diabetically detrimental as any of the others no matter how the health-food addicts strum its praises on their guitars.

Dietetic Foods. Just as many diabetics erroneously believe sweeteners like fructose and sorbitol need not be counted on their diet, they also have the notion that special dietetic foods can be ingested as freely as water and air. Not so! "Dietetic," when used on food labels, has a very precise, ADA-defined meaning. To quote the ADA Exchange Lists, "It means that something has been changed or replaced. It may have less salt, less fat or less sugar. It does not mean that the food is sugar-free or calorie-free."

Monetarily they are a long way from free. In fact, they

sometimes cost twice what their regular nondietetic counterparts cost. And what do you get for these megaprices? A study by Irene M. Wunschel and Bagher M. Sheikholislam of the University of California at Davis revealed that while the amount of carbohydrate in dietetic candy and cookies was less than in regular candy and cookies, the calories and fat were greater. Preserves, syrups, puddings, gelatin, and ice cream rated better in terms of reducing the things a diabetic needs reduced (calories, carbohydrates, fats), but the price differential was significantly greater. Their conclusion was, "In most instances, the consumer receives little or no nutritional benefit from the higher cost of the dietetic product. Indeed, the use of dietetic products may replace foods with important nutrient content. . . . The most beneficial intake is one derived from a wide variety of ordinary foods."

The ADA considers only some dietetic foods useful for diabetics: "Those that contain 20 calories or less per serving may be eaten up to three times a day as free foods."

Shaking Salt

Dr. Andrew Lewin, deputy director of the Hypertension Detection Program at Cedars-Sinai Medical Center in Los Angeles and director of Pressure Partners, a medical program to help patients lower their blood pressure, believes that most Americans are salt addicts, consuming ten to twenty grams of sodium per day. Though health professionals can't agree, the maximum safe level is more like two or three grams a day. (A level teaspoon of salt contains 2.3 grams of sodium; a four-ounce bag of potato chips has about one gram.)

So what if we use too much salt? So a lot. It contributes to high blood pressure, or hypertension, as it's medically called. Studies have revealed that cultures in which the most salt is consumed have the highest rate of hypertension, which is a result of increased water retention in the body. Too much salt also causes swelling of the tissues (edema), which decreases the amount of oxygen they receive, and this in turn can bring a variety of problems associated with circulation.

The "so what" of all this for diabetics is pretty obvious. The problems salt aggravates are many of the same problems diabetes aggravates. Nobody needs double aggravation.

Maturity-onset diabetics who are moving toward (or already into) the high-incidence-of-hypertension years have a particular need to cut back on their salt. But it's a good idea for young diabetics to begin with the basic good-health habit of salt reduction at an early age on the ounce-of-prevention theory. Dr. Lewin believes reducing salt intake will possibly prevent high blood pressure in susceptible persons.

Since everyone under stress is advised to reduce salt in order to avoid the physical stress of water retention, it is only logical that every diabetic, who carries around the built-in stresses of this disease, wouldn't want to add to them with a salt load. If you want to reduce the salt in your diet, here are some tips from Pressure Partners.

1. Learn to distinguish those foods that are high or low in sodium.
2. Read labels carefully to determine the sodium content of processed foods.
3. Avoid processed foods, since they generally contain relatively higher amounts of sodium than their natural or frozen counterparts.
4. Avoid snack foods and restaurant fast foods, which are high in sodium, particularly if you know you have high blood pressure.
5. Find a market that stocks low-sodium products if you have been placed on a sodium-restricted diet.
6. Bring out the natural flavor of foods without using table salt by adding lemon juice, curry powder, honey, herbs, spices, wines, and fruit juices.
7. Use onion and garlic to perk up flavors naturally.

8. Develop your own spice shaker to use at the table in lieu of salt. The shaker may contain onion powder, garlic powder, paprika, pepper, and mixed Italian herbs, or you can create your own blend.

Fortunately, giving up salt is one of the easier give-ups. We discovered this from talking to a dietitian. She said that in her work she was always telling people to take things they enjoyed out of their diets and telling them there was nothing to it, so she decided to try a little self-restricting herself. Since she knew that no one needs additional salt (you get more than you need on a normal diet), she put away her salt shaker and salted nothing at the table. In a few weeks she didn't miss the additional salt at all.

That sounded like a good idea to us, so we both decided to do the salt-shaker boycott. Sure enough, in a few weeks, all craving was gone. In fact, we found we could taste the true flavors of food better without the salt cover-up.

Actually, by giving up salt at the table you may make it unnecessary to have to give it up completely in later years, adding the restriction of a totally sodium-free diet to your already restricted diabetic diet. It's a matter of practicing moderation in order to keep from having to practice abstention.

There have been some recent reports suggesting that sodium may not directly contribute to high blood pressure. Nevertheless, most experts still agree that the 60 million Americans who have high blood pressure should cut back on sodium. Consequently, until evidence to the contrary is clearer, we'll personally continue to consider sodium a dietary criminal.

Le Flour du Mal

White flour is not as much of an active enemy as sugar and salt. Its fault lies not in what it does that's bad but rather in what it doesn't do that's good. The things that are taken out in the refining process are what's mainly good for you in the flour: the bran, which gives you fiber, and the wheat germ, which contains most of the nutrients (B vitamins, vitamin E, iron, and lysine).

Be ye not deceived by the word "enriched." This just means that some of the nutrients that were refined away have been restored. Almost all the trace elements—those appearing in minute quantities—are still gone and, of these, some—such as zinc and chromium—have been considered of special importance for diabetics.

One thing to remember if you decide to switch from white to whole-wheat flour is that whole-wheat flour is a perishable commodity. Try to buy it from a store where you know there's a rapid turnover and where they keep it in a cool place. When you get it home, keep it cool; we usually keep ours in the refrigerator. Often, to be especially sure of freshness, we grind flour ourselves from the wheat berries—but then we're fanatics.

If you can find it, buy stone-ground whole-wheat flour, because fewer of the vitamins are destroyed than in the usual steel-roller milling, which raises the temperature of the wheat. Also, stoneground flour stays fresher longer.

FRIEND OR FOE?

Milk, another white commodity, is not an enemy to most people, but it can be to some. While milk is generally known as the "perfect food" and finds its way onto almost every kind of diabetes exchange list, it does have a few imperfections. For one thing, not everyone has the enzyme (lactase) to digest it. In fact, according to the *Harvard Medical School Health Letter*, 70 to 95 percent of persons of Mediterranean, black-African, and Asian ancestry lack it. Older people, too, sometimes have lost their milk-digesting enzyme. If someone without this enzyme is diagnosed as diabetic and conscientiously tries to consume the milk usually recommended on diabetic diets, it can cause digestive trouble that mimics an irritable colon condition: abdominal cramps, bloating, excessive gas, and diarrhea. If you suspect you may have this problem, your doctor can give you a test to determine if you have a lactase deficiency. People with a lactase deficiency can still enjoy the benefits of milk in such products as ripened cheeses and buttermilk because the lactose has, in effect, been predigested by bacterial cultures. They can also safely drink sweet acidophilus milk which tastes just like regular milk.

All diabetics should also remember that milk does contain a sugar—lactose. An eight-ounce glass gives you the equivalent of a half ounce of sugar, so it can raise your blood sugar. In fact, June uses it to treat hypoglycemia, as do many people in England.

By all means, don't regard milk as an evil product, but do be alert to the disturbances that it can sometimes cause.

FAT CHANCE

As if you didn't have enough of them already, here's another dietary controversy for you to chew on. Is a high level of cholesterol in the bloodstream a risk factor for heart attack and stroke? And does your diet influence that cholesterol level?

Some studies indicate yes on both scores. For example, there was one made in Ethiopia, a country that has a low-fat, high-carbohydrate diet and that boasts a low heart-attack rate. The study was of 130 young adult males—construction workers, college students, and bank employees—living in Addis Ababa. The construction workers ate the traditional diet, mainly whole-grain bread, vegetables, peas, and tea. Only on special occasions did they eat meat. The college students ate what the construction workers ate plus a little more fat from margarine and sausage. The bank clerks added butter, more meat, and a daily egg.

The results? The construction workers' cholesterol averaged 110 milligrams per 100 milliliters, the students averaged 160, and the bank clerks 180. (Young adult male Americans average 200 and at middle age the average rises to 230. In countries where heart attacks are rare the averages don't go over 200.)

Some scientists maintain that cholesterol studies like the preceding are still "inconclusive" and that since the body manufactures its own cholesterol anyway, what you eat isn't all that important. (Scientific studies are, of course, like the Bible. If you search long and hard enough you can usually find a quotation that justifies what you want to do.) We must admit, however, that in our opinion the weight falls on the side of those who *do* consider cholesterol a problem that can and should be avoided, and that changing your diet is the way to avoid it. Dr. Lawrence Power, writing in his syndicated *Food and Fitness* column, sums it up: "Many experts now regard a cholesterol of 200 as the upper limit of normal, a value that the average American exceeds in his twenties and can only reduce by cutting back on his fat-meat intakes and increasing his intake of vegetables and whole-grain foods like bread."

The 1986 report from the National Heart, Lung, and Blood Institute echoes these same sentiments. Their guidelines say that blood cholesterol should be below 200 milligrams and that in the 200 to 239 range a person is at moderate risk for coronary artery disease and at more than 240 at high risk. For those with cholesterol over 240, the Institute recommends treatment first by diet and, if that fails, then by medication.

People at moderate or high risk should also have a test to determine the kinds of cholesterol in their blood. HDLs are high density lipoproteins, the good guys, and LDLs are low density lipoproteins, the bad guys.

That's why we believe that to be on the safe side—always the best side for a diabetic to be on—no matter which diet or combination of diets you follow, you should reduce the foods that tend to raise the level of fats and cholesterol in your bloodstream. To do this, you should replace saturated fats as much as possible with unsaturated fats. It's fairly easy to recognize saturated fats, because they are usually solid or become solid when chilled. Saturated fats are the solid *animal* fats—the marbling that gives prime beef its flavor; the fat of bacon that crisps up so tastily when you fry it; butter, cheese, cream, the fat content in whole milk that gives it its richness; variety meats like sausage and salami; and solid cooking fats like lard.

They are also the vegetable fats coconut oil and palm oil. Although these vegetable fats do not *contain* cholesterol—no vegetable fat does—they do produce cholesterol in the body.

The polyunsaturated fats are the liquid *vegetable* oils like corn, sesame, cottonseed, soybean, and safflower. Fish and poultry also contain more polyunsaturates than beef, lamb, and pork.

There have been recent reports indicating that monounsaturates are as good as or even better than polyunsaturates when it comes to preventing heart disease. One of the reasons for this theory comes from the fact that Italy and Greece—where olive oil, a 77-percent monounsaturate, is universally used—have the lowest rates of heart disease. Other high monounsaturates are canola oil, and a new California entry, avocado oil.

Currently our oils of choice are olive and avocado. The former gives a wonderful flavor to salads and sauces. June prefers the more delicate French olive oil, Barbara, the lustier Italian. In either case, since you don't use much of it, you should get the best, extra virgin (also called double virgin), which is from the first pressing of the olives. The second best is virgin, from the second pressing. We suggest avoiding the misnamed "pure" olive oil, which comes from treating the pressed-out olive pulp with chemicals, and the also misnamed "fine" olive oil, which is actually "pure" olive oil diluted with water.

Despite all of its virtues, olive oil has too pronounced a flavor for all kitchen uses. Avocado oil, we find, is ideal. This versatile oil is water-processed without chemicals or preservatives. It has a *very* high smoke point, which means that on those rare occasions when you fry foods, you can get the oil extremely hot before adding the foods; thus less oil is absorbed into the food. Avocado oil also has only 8.2 calories per gram rather than the 9 calories of most other oils and butter. You can reduce calories and cholesterol in recipes calling for butter by substituting one-half or even two-thirds of the butter with avocado oil. The flavor will still be there because avocado oil has something of a buttery taste itself. Incidentally, it doesn't taste at all like avocados, so even people who don't like avocados will enjoy it. It's also a great little emulsifier so you can easily whip up nice thick salad dressings and mayonnaise with it.

Egg yolks are very high in cholesterol (one large egg yolk contains 252 milligrams). June's doctor hasn't had an egg in twelve years and his cholesterol is 150. But just to keep the controversy alive, we ought to tell you that there are those who say eggs contain lecithin, which negates their cholesterol. (Sigh!) Organ meats such as liver and kidney are extremely high in cholesterol. If you're a liver fancier and feel that giving it up would be a great loss, remember that the liver in animals is a great depository of DDT and other noxious chemicals that might be even more disastrous to your health than cholesterol. If you give up liver and other organ meats, you'll be avoiding these poisons as well as cholesterol.

Shellfish are on the high-cholesterol list, also alas!, but the recent scientific position is that even though shellfish are relatively high in cholesterol, they're so low in saturated fat that even if you're on a low-cholesterol diet you don't have to eliminate them entirely. Oysters, clams, and scallops are the lowest in cholesterol and are the preferred choice. Shrimp, lobster, and crab, although higher in cholesterol, are again, low in saturated fat, so with them too you're okay; but watch the amounts you eat more closely.

Putting Your Fats on a Diet

Cutting down on your fat is of prime importance in reducing cholesterol and also in weight loss. (A gram of fat has more than twice the calories of a gram of protein or carbohydrate!)

Here are a few of the trades we worked out for ourselves to help in fat and cholesterol reduction.

Butter is bad for your cholesterol, but have you ever looked at the label of a carton of soft margarine and seen the chemical concoction that it is? With that many chemicals in one place, who knows how many of them singly or in combination will turn out in later studies to do something dreadful to you? And we know that miscellaneous alien chemicals can be stressors to the body. Fortunately, the authors of the outstanding vegetarian cookbook, *The New Laurel's Kitchen,* have taken care of this problem with their Better-Butter recipe. Better-Butter is not only delicious but it spreads very easily, so you can use less of it.

Better-Butter

1 cup safflower, soy, or corn oil
1 cup butter (two cubes)
2 tablespoons water
2 tablespoons dried skim milk
1/4 teaspoon lecithin
1/2 teaspoon salt

In blender, dissolve salt in water. Add all other ingredients and blend until smooth. Pour into containers and store in refrigerator.

Speaking of using less butter, if you have flavorful homemade bread, you really don't need butter or anything else on it. In France, where they don't worry much about fat and cholesterol, only about taste, they never use butter on bread except at breakfast.

The amount of butter and other fats you use in cooking can be vastly reduced without adversely affecting flavor. We now usually use only about one-third the amount of fat called for in a recipe. For example, when you sauté onions to soften them, if you cover the pan and let them steam you need to use ony a half or a third as much fat as called for.

Steaming vegetables is another way to decrease the amount of fat you use in food preparation. We find that they retain so much flavor with this method that we can sprinkle on a few herbs and/or parsley or maybe, as in the case of green beans, spread on a little mustard or other nonfat seasoning. If you do put butter on steamed vegetables, you'll find you can use less, because they won't be all wet and soggy and the butter will cling better. Another plus is that steaming retains vitamins.

An air popper for popcorn allows you to eliminate totally all the gratuitous and invisible fat you get when popcorn is cooked in the usual way with oil. Incidentally, let us praise popcorn. Any product a diabetic can have three cups of for one starch exchange has to have something going for it. *And* it's full of fiber!

Always use nonfat milk. Low-fat milk is a snare and a delusion, because each cup contains five grams of fat. When you realize that whole milk has eight grams, low-fat isn't that much of a change. Nonfat has less than one gram, or none.

Always use nonfat yogurt. With nonfat yogurt, you have the basis for fat-free salad dressings. Here are a few of our favorite combinations:

Mustard Yogurt. Flavor the amount of nonfat yogurt you need for dressing with a bit of prepared mustard. We prefer Dijon, but any brand you like will serve the purpose.

Oriental Yogurt. Add garlic powder and a small amount of soy sauce or tamari and ginger to the yogurt.

Herbed Yogurt. Add any herbs you particularly like. One combination we favor is tarragon, basil, and chervil. For an Italian touch, use oregano, basil, and garlic. With spinach salad try tarragon, garlic, a dash of artificial sweetener or fructose balanced off with a little vinegar to taste, and artificial bacon bits.

Minted Yogurt. Add a hint—but *just* a hint—of fresh mint. This is particularly good with fruit salads.

Incidentally, salad dressings without oil and sugar are now appearing on market shelves. Watch for them.

Yogurt is also excellent on fruit, and it's marvelous on soups and in vegetables. Purée fruit in the blender and add it to yogurt for a terrific dessert. Or thin the dessert down with milk and blend it some more and you have the delicious fruit-yogurt drink known as kefir.

Experiment with yogurt; it has infinite possibilities, and this goes without even mentioning all the good that health-food addicts believe the acidophilus bacilli do for your intestinal flora.

Sour cream is normally a fat-a-thon, but you can make a commendable substitute with a quarter cup of buttermilk blended with three-quarters cup of cottage cheese. Also try this "sour cream" on a baked potato with lots of chopped parsley and chives or green-onion tops.

You can blend cottage cheese alone to make an imitation cream cheese. Barbara, who is a lox-and-bagel-and-cream-cheese fan, chops up bits of smoked salmon into the cottage cheese blend and spreads it on a bagel—which, incidentally, is a good fat-free kind of bread.

One of the big losses on a low-fat diet is the loss of most—and certainly the best—cheeses because of their high, mostly saturated-fat content: eight to nine grams of fat per ounce or two high-fat Meat Exchanges. In addition, you have to be careful about their sodium content; the processed ones have more than the natural ones. Actually, though, not all cheeses are gone. Most of you are allowed a certain amount of the reduced-fat varieties now readily available or those, like part-skim-milk mozzarella and Muenster, that have only five to six grams of fat per ounce.

We have a philosophy that we would rather have a very small amount of an excellent cheese we really want in a dish we're cooking rather than compromise the taste by using low-fat substitutions. We often order good cheeses by mail, package them in tiny pieces, and freeze them. If sealed in a moisture-proof airtight plastic bag, they keep for months.

The general guidelines are to eat cheese sparingly or in moderation. To achieve this, you need to have specific dietary information about whatever ones you choose. The best source for this is a table published in the November/December 1990 issue of *Diabetes Self-Management* (150 West 22nd Street, New York, NY 10011; phone 1-212-989-0200 for purchase; $3.00 plus $2.50 shipping).

When it comes to eggs, what we generally do is leave half the yolks out in scrambled eggs or omelets and in most recipes calling for eggs. (This usually means adding extra eggs, because if you're using fewer yolks you need more whites.)

There are also a number of egg substitutes on the market. If you decide to use these, Dr. Anderson suggests you select the ones with fewer than two hundred calories per cup.

We discover new fat- and cholesterol-avoidance every day. And, of course, we are not alone. Manufacturers have long been working in their labs to develop a fat substitute, literally a nonfat fat. Two such substances are now being used in commercial products: NutraSweet's Simplesse and Procter & Gamble's Olestra. Simplesse is a low-fat fat not suitable for cooking. It is composed of whey protein from milk or egg whites (beware if you have an allergy to either) and replaces twenty-seven calories of fat with four calories of protein. Olestra is mainly sucrose and vegetable oil bonded into molecules too large to digest. It can be used in cooking.

So stay on your guard until these dietary miracles come to pass. Use your own ingenuity in playing the low-fat game. It's a challenge and, in its own way, fun—something like doing the *New York Times* crossword puzzle. If you get into the spirit of it, you'll soon develop your own set of tricks to eliminate fat and cholesterol and the alleged cardiovascular problems that go along with them.

Control through Control

And here's a final tip on controlling your cholesterol. One of the best ways to do it is through keeping your diabetes in good control. According to Dr. Julio Rosenstock of the University of Texas Health Science Center, doing so will "lower a patient's plasma cholesterol, low-density lipoprotein cholesterol [the bad cholesterol], and triglyceride levels."

VEGETARIANISM

Vegetarianism, or at least cutting back on red meat in the diet, is becoming a way of eating for people with all kinds of health problems, as well as for those who have no health problems and want to keep it that way. Many young people are adopting vegetarianism as an act of conscience or, some say, as an act of hostility against their parents! If, for whatever reason, you lean toward a vegetarian diet, your diabetes won't prevent you from following that inclination. Whether you follow the standard Exchange List diet, the HCF diet, or Bernstein's method, it's possible for you to be a vegetarian, although you will have to take certain precautions and make certain adjustments.

If you want to be a lacto-ovo vegetarian on the HCF diet, you'll have to make it nonfat lacto-egg-white-o (or egg-substitute-o). To be a vegan (one who consumes neither eggs or milk products nor meat, poultry, or fish) on HCF would be a natural. On Bernstein's plan you couldn't be a strict vegan, but it would be possible to be a lacto-ovo, meeting your protein need on eggs, cheese, soybean products, and nuts, and using the lower-carbohydrate vegetables. With the standard diabetes diet you could be a lacto-ovo or, with a great deal of tightrope walking, a vegan.

If you want to adopt either kind of vegetarian diet, you have to study and learn a great deal. Fortunately, there are excellent books to refer to. Marion Franz, R.D., in *Exchanges for All Occasions,* has an entire chapter called "If You Want to Be a Vegetarian," in which she provides a list of special vegetarian exchanges.

We also heartily recommend *The New Laurel's Kitchen.* Its philosophy is beautiful, the recipes delicious and totally unlike some of the strange ersatz guck sometimes served up in the name of vegetarianism, and the scientific dietary information impeccable and understandable. *The New Laurel's Kitchen*, again unlike many vegetarian cookbooks, is against the use of excessive amounts of sweets and fats, which makes it especially good for diabetics. We also recommend and use ourselves *Sunset Vegetarian Cooking*, which includes a nutritional analysis of each recipe; *The Vegetarian Gourmet; The Vegetarian Epicure* and *The Vegetarian Epicure: Book Two;* and *Greene on Greens*.

As more and more people become interested in vegetarianism, whether for moral, health, or economic reasons, more and more good vegetarian cookbooks are bound to appear. Watch for them, and especially for ones written for diabetics.

THE FRUIT, THE WHOLE FRUIT, AND NOTHING BUT THE FRUIT

Over the years June has given up drinking fruit juice in any circumstances except to counteract insulin reactions. She found that the juice shot her blood sugar up in a way that the fruit itself didn't seem to. This discovery was later confirmed by Dr. Lawrence Power in his *Food and Fitness* newspaper column: "Fruit juice can give your system a jolt. . . . Recent studies by nutrition scientists reveal that a six-ounce glass of any natural fruit juice will sharply increase blood-sugar levels to a peak." In nondiabetics, he explained, this can cause the body to overreact, resulting in hypoglycemia with its old familiar episodes of shaking, sweating, and anxiety. We all know what a sugar jolt like that does to a diabetic.

This blood-sugar peaking rarely occurs after eating the whole fruit; apparently the pulp slows down the action. We've also noticed that for snacks on the HCF diet, Dr. Anderson recommends a piece of whole-wheat bread or some rye crackers in conjunction with fresh fruit. The fiber of the bread exchange slows the fruit down even further.

Incidentally, if you're in the habit of drinking orange juice made from a frozen concentrate, you might be interested in Dr. Power's description of that product: "Frozen orange juice is really a concentrate of sugar from the orange. . . . Oranges by the truckload are dumped on a conveyer belt, scrubbed clean, split and reamed, and the juice filtered to remove pulp (and thus any nutrient contribution the pulp might make) and seeds. It then enters a holding tank, where it is heated to kill any germs, and vacuum-evaporated to a thick, orange-colored sugar syrup." And that's what you defrost, dilute, and drink.

VITAMIN AND MINERAL SUPPLEMENTS

We always wear kid gloves when entering the vitamin/mineral supplement arena. No health subject is more fraught with controversy and contradiction. Dr. Ron Brown, our former Sugar-Free Center dietitian who is now an M.D., has what we have come to think is the soundest advice. If you have no known vitamin deficiencies, your best bet is to get all your vitamins and minerals from your good-and-healthy balanced diabetic diet. But just as a safety net, Ron advises one multivitamin tablet a day.

This kind of uniform one-a-day prescription does not, of course, apply to all people of all ages and sexes. Women, in particular, usually need extra calcium and/or iron. The recommended daily dietary allowance (RDA) of calcium for women is 800 to 1,000 mg., but growing girls and pregnant and lactating women need at least 1,200 to 1,400 mg. a day. Post-menopausal women not receiving estrogen should have at least 1,500 mg.

daily. (To get that amount, you'd need the equivalent of two quarts of milk.) As you can see, what supplements to take and the amounts is another of those manifold check-with-your-doctor activities.

In spite of our cautious attitude, we want to make you aware that new studies are showing that diabetics may suffer from vitamin C deficiency, and supplements of 1,500 mg. a day may improve their A_{1c} tests. Also, high E (1,000 I.U. a day) may do the same thing. These two vitamins (antioxidants) are also thought to protect against heart disease and cancer.

Two trace minerals—zinc and chromium—have been touted by many of the antiestablishment diet and health books and magazines as having blood-sugar-lowering benefits for diabetics. The scientific evidence on which these claims are based has to do with the following facts: zinc plays a role in carbohydrate metabolism, chromium deficiency can raise blood glucose, and chromium supplementation improves glucose tolerance in some older people. However, we can find no large-scale studies that give conclusive results on these two minerals for diabetics. We therefore favor waiting for definitive evidence of their benefits before loading up on supplements.

Another supplement craze has been fish oil, in particular the omega-3 fatty acids found in cold-water fish like salmon, herring, sardines, mackerel, tuna, cod, shrimp, lobster, crab, and the like. Researchers found that omega-3s lowered cholesterol and triglycerides and removed some of the risk of heart attack and stroke. More recently, however, warnings have come out about the possible dangers of high-dosage supplements of omega-3. In fact, they are not recommended by the American Diabetes Association or the American Heart Association, and the latest indication that they can be dangerous is that the FDA has ordered manufacturers to stop further distribution. The best advice we can give you is to eat cold-water fish at least twice a week. But you should be doing that anyway: fish is a very healthy food.

CHEMICALS

June became very conscious of chemicals in food during her headache years because many chemicals, notably MSG and nitrates or nitrites, were known to cause headaches. Since a headache is a common symptom of low blood sugar, a diabetic who doesn't want to have to deal with confusing body signals would naturally want to avoid headache-producing substances. On top of that, these chemicals have other side effects that are detrimental to your health.

Take the "flavor enhancer" MSG—or, rather, *don't* take it if you can avoid it. When you read labels you'll find it's in almost every processed food. Besides producing headaches in susceptible individuals, it also produces dizziness, nasal congestion, and general feelings of malaise among others. But that's not the worst of it. MSG is mono*sodium* glutamate. That sodium is the same old sodium that does you wrong in salt, and it does you wrong in exactly the same ways.

Nitrates and nitrites are suspected cancer producers, and cancer does not improve diabetes. Actually, you have a double reason for avoiding nitrates and nitrites. They are usually found in things like bacon, sausage, hot dogs, and lunch meats, which are also full of another item high on the diabetes nix list: fat.

Besides these known enemy chemicals in food, there are hundreds of unknowns that are currently on the Federal Drug Administration's GRAS (Generally Regarded as Safe) list. Remember, though, a goodly number of the chemicals that are now forbidden in food were once Generally Regarded as Safe by the FDA. A chemical is like an accused person in our system of justice: innocent until proven guilty. To be on the safe side, we prefer to shun as many of these potential criminals as possible. This usually means reading the label, rejecting the product, sighing heavily, and deciding to fix the food from scratch, using fresh ingredients.

Unfortunately, even fresh ingredients are suspect these days, what with wide use of chemical fertilizers and pesticides. Health-food stores advertise their vegetables, fruits, and grains as "organically grown" and claim that they are free from all harmful chemicals. We've read several studies, however, showing that these fruits and vegetables often come from the same bins in the very same wholesale-produce markets as those you find in the supermarket. The only thing that's different about them is the higher price. That's why we shop mostly at farmer's markets or grow our own fruits and vegetables (see pages 104–7).

One important change is the Nutrition Labeling and Education Act of 1990, mandating easier-to-understand nutrition labels on most prepared foods by May 1993. The FDA must also define those ambiguous terms *natural*, *fresh*, and *organic*, which have been used for years to trick us into purchasing items that, if the truth be known, we would rather not consume. We must pray now that these admirable intentions will not be thwarted by special interests, as happened when the U.S. Department of Agriculture was pressured to stop publication and distribution of its pamphlet called *The Eating-Right Food Pyramid*.

CAFFEINE

Diabetic dietitian Meg Gaekle calls coffee "the last vestige of diabetic freedom." So it is! This nice, comforting beverage is a mood elevator well known for its ability literally to wake you up and make you more alert. It has now even been scientifically substantiated that coffee decreases fatigue and makes you think more clearly. No wonder we naturally gravitate toward it.

So what's wrong with drinking coffee? The psychoactive drug in coffee is, of course, caffeine. And over the years we've all heard that caffeine does terrible things to your body. It's been accused of causing heart disease, high blood pressure, high blood cholesterol levels, and different forms of cancer, including pancreatic—all the things diabetics in particular don't need.

But now, thanks to large-scale scientific studies by qualified researchers, caffeine is losing its evil image. It's now being reported that you're safe from those reputed damaging physical effects if you keep your consumption of caffeine to no more than two or three cups a day. This is certainly welcome news, because coffee is *free* in the diabetic sense of the word. And, of course, so is tea, which also contains caffeine. So are sugar-free soft drinks, many of which also contain caffeine. The following chart from the FDA shows the caffeine content of a five-ounce serving of hot beverages and a twelve-ounce serving of soft drinks, as well as other sources of caffeine. Two hundred milligrams of caffeine a day appear to be a safe amount for most people (those with heart arrhythmias are an exception).

Decaffeinated coffee: 2–5 mg.
Percolated coffee: 40–170 mg.
Drip-brewed coffee: 60–185 mg.
Instant coffee: 30–120 mg.
Brewed tea: 20–115 mg.
Instant tea: 25–50 mg.
Cocoa: 2–20 mg.
Many soft drinks: 30–55 mg.
Weight-loss drugs, diuretics: 100–200 mg.
Pain relievers: 30–100 mg.
Cold/allergy remedies: 15–30 mg.

What if you overdo on caffeine? It can make you very nervous and jumpy as well as create a bad case of insomnia. And the amount of coffee that you can drink without experiencing adverse symptoms is a very individual matter. Much depends on whether you're a regular consumer. If you regularly drink 250 milligrams a day (two to three cups), caffeine will have no significant effect on your blood pressure, heart rate, respiration, metabolic rate, blood glucose concentration, or cholesterol level. But if you haven't had any for a week or two, the effects may be more pronounced.

Speaking of blood glucose levels, coffee does cause blood sugar to rise somewhat. It also aggravates ulcers, and, most seriously, it does "hasten the excretion of calcium from the body, which could increase the risk of osteoporosis," according to the *Johns Hopkins Medical Letter* of March 1991. Another negative: since caffeine is a drug, it has withdrawal symptoms, mainly headache and fatigue. It takes about a week to lose these symptoms. (Don't take a caffeine-containing over-the-counter painkiller when giving up caffeine!)

Our compromise with coffee drinking, in view of all this new research, is to grind together half regular and half decaffeinated beans. Also, there is the alternative of herb teas, although these are not always harmless. Some ginseng teas have up to 85 percent sugar, and this may not be on the label. Above all, don't let anyone tell you that you can cure diabetes with any kind of herb tea.

ALCOHOL

We once heard a wise dietitian speaking at a diabetes seminar. She told her fellow dietitians that when a diabetic patient asks if it's all right to have a cocktail before dinner or a glass or two of wine with dinner, it's not much help to say, "You'll have to ask your doctor about that." It's not much help, she said, because we all know full well what the doctor will say. The doctor who's a teetotaler will say, "Absolutely not. No alcohol at all. Not a drop." The doctor who's *not* a teetotaler will say, "I don't think a cocktail or a glass of wine will hurt you."

So what is a diabetic supposed to do when it comes to drinking? We suggest looking at the facts and making an intelligent decision based on your own lifestyle. Actually, that's what we suggest in all areas of diabetes care.

It's an undeniable fact that alcohol contains calories and, in some cases, carbohydrate. If weight is a problem, as it is with many maturity-onset diabetics who are not insulin-dependent, drinking can augment that problem. If you *do* drink, you have to count the alcohol as part of your diet. If you're already on a low-calorie diet to lose weight, then cutting back on the food in order to add the drink can cause you to wind up with truly slim pickings at mealtime. For example, if you're on a 1,400-calorie diet and you drink one and a half ounces of scotch, that uses up 108 of your calories.

Not only that, but the calories you get from alcohol are like those in sugar—empty. That is to say, they contain nothing that's good for you. A comedian once suggested that they should produce vitamin gin so you could build yourself up while you tear yourself down. As a matter of fact, it has been seriously suggested that there should be additives to alcoholic beverages, but the government won't allow it, probably on the theory that it would only encourage people to drink more—hardly a national goal.

In fitting alcohol into the day's food calculations with the Exchange Lists, you count it as a fat. An ounce and a half of hard liquor is two Fat Exchanges. A four-ounce glass of dry wine is also two Fat Exchanges. Beer is one Starch/Bread plus two Fat Exchanges because it contains carbohydrates as well as alcohol.

Drinking is not recommended on the HCF diet, because it seems to cause a rise in triglycerides. Dr. Anderson is realistic enough to know that his patients sometimes do drink (one of his veteran patients even goes so far as to stow away an occasional six-pack). He figures that if the drinking isn't excessive and the patient is neither overweight nor high in triglycerides, then drinking doesn't completely destroy the virtues of the HCF diet.

For someone following Bernstein's high-protein, high-fat plan, alcohol presents a particular problem because it can keep proteins from being converted to glucose. Since this diet uses protein rather than carbohydrate as the main source of glucose, an alcoholic drink at mealtime can be dangerous.

Furthermore, alcohol is risky for diabetics taking either insulin or oral hypoglycemics because it can interact adversely with them.

Another problem with alcohol for diabetics who are overweight is that it tends to lower inhibitions, and your formerly well-controlled hand may start straying toward the cocktail snacks and popping them into your mouth. Therefore, you get calories upon calories—those of the alcohol plus those in the snacks.

For insulin takers, on the other hand, the danger with alcohol is compounded in several respects, most having to do with hypoglycemia. First—and this is true for all diabetics, according to Dr. Leo P. Krall—if you eat while drinking, alcohol will push your blood sugar up; but if you *don't* eat while drinking, alcohol can lower your blood sugar. So you can get in trouble in both directions.

Here's another hypoglycemic possibility. To keep blood sugar normal, the body can manufacture sugar from its stored animal starch (glycogen), which is called gluconeogenesis. Alcohol blocks gluconeogenesis. Insulin also blocks release of glucose from the liver. So an insulin-dependent diabetic who has not eaten for a while—thus depleting the body's glycogen supply—and who then drinks alcohol is in severe danger of experiencing a blood-sugar plummet to the insulin-reaction level.

If, in addition, alcohol makes you forget to eat at the time you need to, you could become slurring of speech and staggering of gait and perhaps even pass out. The average policeman—in fact, the average anybody—would be likely to consider you a common drunk, as they like to call them, and treat you accordingly. The treatment of a common drunk is not the kind of treatment that brings about a raising of the blood sugar.

Alcohol also reduces the body's ability to fight infection, and since diabetics are already more susceptible to infection it's unwise to further reduce the defenses.

Oh, yes, and there's always the liver damage that accompanies long-term excessive drinking. But then we aren't here discussing long-term excessive drinking for diabetics. *Nobody* condones that.

When you come right down to it, you're probably getting the answer here that you get from a doctor who will take an occasional drink. Done intelligently in moderation, it's not ghastly for you and your diabetes. However, although we both drink (intelligently, in moderation) and consider a glass of wine something that embellishes a meal, we freely acknowledge that it's better for a diabetic not to drink—just as it's better for a nondiabetic not to drink. It's an alien chemical that you're throwing into your system, and alien chemicals in the body cause stress. Besides, we get enough alien chemicals that we can't avoid these days without adding those we can.

If you want to give up alcohol, it might help if you realize that it is possible that your desire for a drink is more a desire to put something into your mouth—a need for oral gratification that a soft drink will satisfy as well as a hard one. Not that we're particularly recommending soft drinks for diabetics—not even artificially sweetened ones—but we *do* recommend that you try to find something other than alcohol. Possibly it could be something like one of the new mineral waters with a twist of lemon or a dash of bitters at cocktail time. Or if you want to have a drink with very little alcohol but with lots of putting in the mouth and swallowing, you could try a spritzer made with a small amount of wine and a large amount of club soda or mineral water.

Mineral water, incidentally, can have several advantages. You are, after all, drinking *something,* so you don't feel odd or different or left out when others are swilling away. (We've often found that with many of the restrictions of the diabetic diet, giving up certain things is not the hardest part. The hardest part is feeling you're not doing what everyone else is doing. It's a pity we all have these tuggings toward conformity, but we do seem to.) Then, too, a mineral water such as Perrier is usually as expensive as an alcoholic drink so you won't feel you're incurring the wrath of the waiter or bartender by taking up the space of a paying customer without buying anything.

Mineral water is also now very much the drink of those beautiful people who want to stay slim and alert and who shun anything alcoholic, sugary, or chemical-laden. And, finally, there's the simple fact that drinking pure water is excellent for your general health. Most of us simply don't drink enough of it. If we can incorporate water drinking into a social ritual, it's all to the good.

One delightful new development on the drinking scene is the arrival of alcohol-free wines such as Ariél (from California) and Hans Barth (from Germany). These wines actually have less alcohol than that contained naturally in orange juice. (We didn't know there was *any* alcohol in orange juice. Maybe that's why so many Type I diabetics insist on drinking orange juice to bring up their blood sugar when we all know that glucose tablets and even, according to the Glycemic Index, mashed potatoes bring it up faster.) A special advantage for people on a weight-loss program is that these wines have half the calories of regular wine.

Though low in calories, the wines are high in quality—and cost (seventeen dollars a bottle in restaurants). Ariél offers brut champagne as well as white, rosé, and red wine. A glass (three ounces) is five grams of carbohydrate and twenty-six calories. Hans Barth has a very dry Riesling. It is even "freer," with only four grams of carbohydrate and fifteen calories per four-ounce glass.

More recently the market has been flooded with alcohol-free beers. We counted thirteen varieties in a local liquor store. They're called *malt beverages,* and the alcohol content is usually .5 percent. Domestically there is Miller's *Sharp's,* Pabst's *Cheers,* Anheuser-Busch's *O'Doul's,* and so on. Imported labels include Heineken's *Buckler,* Guinness's *Kaliber,* and several from Germany. The main diabetic drawback is the carbohydrate content, which is between eleven and fifteen grams for a twelve-ounce bottle. Calories run about fifty to seventy per bottle. In taste, we decided they resemble very light ales, usually with a slight hint of sweetness. Our favorites were Buckler, O'Doul's, and St. Pauli Girl.

If these wines and beers prove successful, it's almost certain that this happy trend will continue and other wineries will offer alcohol-free selections.

SMOKING—THE UNBEARABLE

Okay folks, brace yourselves for a rant. We are unalterably opposed to smoking. In fact, we hate it. Fortunately, we are not alone in our intolerant attitude. While drinking doctors may approve of an occasional cocktail or glass of wine for diabetics, even a chain-smoking doctor (and there are fewer of them every day—you might say they're a dying breed) will not give a diabetic the go-ahead on smoking.

Smoking has been called the number-one preventable cause of death. Whatever verbal pussyfooting the tobacco industry engages in, the fact is you run a hugely greater risk of getting chronic bronchitis, emphysema, and lung cancer if you smoke. Unfortunately, just because the gods have chosen to plague you with diabetes does not mean you have a built-in immunity to other diseases.

As a diabetic, however, you have special reasons not to smoke. Smoking causes a narrowing of the blood vessels and this makes you even more susceptible to those cardiovascular problems that are already lurking about ready to pounce on a diabetic. Because of this blood-vessel constriction, smoking also further complicates another complication of diabetes—poor circulation. As you know, poor circulation can help bring about such diabetic delights as gangrenous toes.

And are you ready for another negative effect of smoking? This is a greater risk for retinitis, the condition that can lead to blindness. Blood-vessel constriction leads to a lessened blood flow, which in turn causes a decrease in oxygen content of tissues (hypoxia), which ups the chances for developing that blindness-inducing retinitis.

We've also noticed that smokers always seem to be nervous and twitchy. Does the nicotine make them so or are they just nervous and twitchy waiting for their next nicotine fix? We don't know, but these nervous twitchers are obviously under stress. (They also put others around them under the stress of having to watch them.) And stress is exactly what we're trying to deliver diabetics from.

If you gather from the above that we're against smoking for diabetics, you gather correctly. In fact, if you're a smoker and you ever visit either of us, please check your cigarettes at the door.

If you don't smoke, don't start. It's not sophisticated, it's stupid. It is, as former HEW Secretary Joseph Califano called it, "slow-motion suicide." It's also said by some to be a harder habit to break than heroin. If you already have the vile habit, do whatever you have to do to break it, even to the point of paying for a service, such as Smokenders or Schick, to help you. (In some areas the American Cancer Society has free smoking-stopping programs.)

End of rant.

MARIJUANA

Our first objection to marijuana is the same as our objection to smoking. After all, you do smoke it—unless, of course, you make it into Alice B. Toklas brownies, in which case our objection is the same as our objection to sugar. In addition to that, marijuana has the inhibition-reducing and judgment-suspending qualities of alcohol, the problems of which we've already discussed. It also shares with alcohol a tendency to weaken the body's immune system. In addition to *that,* with marijuana usually comes the munchies, prompting you, almost uncontrollably, to eat everything in sight, and there goes the diet.

In addition to *that,* marijuana may cause high blood sugar by breaking down and releasing the body's stored glycogen. In addition to *that,* it's illegal. And, finally, in addition to *that,* it's still an unknown commodity as far as what it does to your long-range health. Those who maintain that it's less detrimental than alcohol may well be wrong. It may merely be that alcohol has been used so extensively and its effects have been studied for such a long period of time that we're more aware of the damage it does. It may be years before the ill effects of long-term marijuana use are discovered, and then it may be too late.

When you do all of this addition, it's clear that marijuana should be subtracted from any diabetic's list of drugs.

COCAINE

At first we weren't even going to bring up the subject of cocaine. After all, what person in his or her right mind who already has one expensive habit—diabetes—would want to take up another? (We once heard cocaine defined as nature's way of telling you that you have too much money.) But, according to statistics, there are *many* people not in their right minds. An estimated five million Americans are regular cocaine users and thirty million have tried it at least once. Therefore, we'll present you with some of the potential hazards of cocaine use.

Cocaine has been proven to cause nasal passage damage including loss of the sense of smell, constriction of blood vessels, quick rise in blood pressure, angina, irregular heartbeat, a rupturing of the aorta, heart attacks, strokes (both the paralyzing and killing variety), atherosclerotic heart disease, drowning from a sudden accumulation of fluid in the lungs, liver damage, seizures, tremors, delirium, psychosis, impotence, and, in pregnancy, fetal damage or death, and infant abnormalities such as low birth weight and a panoply of neurobehavioral disorders. Is that enough for you? If not, try death, which can occur during your first experiment with the drug.

CHAPTER 4

Diet: The Art of the Matter

It always confounds us when we hear diabetics talk about how difficult it is to stay on the diet because they neither want to cook two separate and different meals nor (horror of horrors) impose the diabetic diet on the rest of the family. You'd think the diet was something as grotesque as the one diabetic world traveler Jerry Evens described as his standard fare on one exotic excursion: barbecued monkeys, iguana tails, manioc root, and fried green bananas.

The standard diabetic diet is nothing more than a perfectly balanced nutritious meal plan—the kind of meal plan every person who cares about health should be following. The HCF diet is to our minds an even more healthful variation on that theme. If you get your family onto the diabetic diet, each member should leave a little note of gratitude next to your plate at mealtime because, thanks to your disease, you've made them all aware of the proper way to eat for vitality, longevity, and an attractive appearance.

As June says, with passionate vehemence, "I wish to God I had lived with a diabetic when I was young." As it was, she didn't learn a thing about good nutrition until she was forty-five and diagnosed as diabetic. Who knows, had she known about good nutrition all her life she might never have had to be diagnosed as diabetic. And who knows how many maladies *you* are keeping away from the family door by the "imposition of your diet."

THE JOY OF COOKING

You may feel that you can't fit "scratch" cooking into a schedule already crammed with diabetes activities. But stay. Cooking not only provides the additive-free, nutritious food you need to maintain optimum health and diabetes control; it also can be a mental-health booster and stress reducer in itself.

The writer John Irving says, "If you are careful, if you use good ingredients and you don't take any short cuts, then you can usually cook something very good. Sometimes it is the only worthwhile product you can salvage from a day. With writing, I find, you can have all the right ingredients, give plenty of time and care and still get nothing. Also true of love. Cooking, therefore, keeps a person who tries hard sane."

Also true of diabetes. How often have you tried hard and still come up with a 250 blood sugar? Cooking keeps you sane, but only if you don't go about it insanely. If you attack your cooking in a frenzy, trying to get it over with as quickly as possible, you'll build up stresses that even the most perfect diet will have trouble counteracting. Working quietly and concentrating on what you're doing makes cooking creative, enjoyable, and sanity promoting.

A MULCH BETTER WAY TO GARDEN

One very good cook of our acquaintance says that the secret of cooking is to get the best, freshest ingredients you can and do as little to them as possible. The ideal way to get those ingredients is to grow them yourself in a vegetable garden.

For that you need the space and time. We know that not everyone has the space, but no matter how busy you are, you have the time, if you garden Ruth Stout's way. Ruth Stout was the author of *The No-Work Garden Book*, which is unfortunately now out of print (and Ruth is now no longer gardening in this world, but her legacy lingers on). Prior to reading Ruth's book we used to sweat and strain and hoe and weed (and weed and weed and weed) and wind up with semi-paltry harvests. Now, thanks to her, we have bountiful crops with so little work it's embarrassing. Here's how you do it. Spade up your garden for the last time in your whole life. Call up a local feed store and ask them if they have any old rained-on straw or hay that they want to sell for cheap. They almost always do. Buy enough to cover your garden to a depth of six to eight inches. If you buy too much that's okay because you can put it around other things like flowers and trees.

Push aside the hay or straw and dig a hole and put in your plant in the normal way. We water them deeply with water containing vitamin B to keep the plant from getting shocked by the move. Then you bring the straw back up around it so the plant's head is sticking up. And that's about all there is to it. Ruth thinks you hardly ever need to water again, but since we're in Southern California, where it almost never rains in the summer (and lately in any other season, either), we do water when the plants start to look droopy. We don't water much, though. In fact, the reason we first decided to give Ruth's method a try was that we were having a terrible drought and wanted to conserve as much water as possible.

Regarding seeds, Ruth has you plant them and cover them with a light layer of sawdust or loose straw until the plants grow up enough to get the straw pulled up around them. Should a stray weed have the audacity to grow up through the straw, just throw a handful of straw on top and it will never be seen again. The tiny bit of work you do in the garden—mainly harvesting your crop—is accomplished without even getting your shoes dirty or muddy. The straw is quite clean and brushes off easily.

What to plant? Whatever appeals to you and grows well in your area. The nursery people will be able to tell you the best thrivers. But don't forget the herbs. They'll enhance every dish and are freebies for diabetics.

Each year the mulch rots down to enrich the soil, so you don't need fertilizers. And according to Ruth, even the hallowed compost pile is unnecessary.

Ruth confesses that with her method you do have one problem: you get such a huge crop of vegetables you have trouble giving them away. We've used her method for only one year, and already we've had that problem!

So now if you have the space, you have no excuse not to have the most fantastically flavorful vegetables you've ever eaten. Your success may inspire you to put in a few fruit trees as well. The food-gardening momentum tends to build. If you don't have much space, try gardening in containers. If you don't have even that much space, put some herbs in pots. One of our fondest memories is of the summer we got to spend a couple of weeks in a house that some friends of ours had restored in the south of France in Ménerbes, just up the hill from the area Peter Mayle is making famous in his books. There was no yard and no terrace on which to grow things, but there was a pot of fresh basil on the kitchen sink, and we snipped leaves from that and put them in and on everything we cooked for a wonderful Provençal flavor. Start creating your own herbaceous memories.

THE FARMER IN THE PARKING LOT

If you have no place for a garden and no terrace for containers, there's a new trend starting that you should look out for. It can be your dietary salvation: farmer's markets. In the last couple of years they've been springing up all over the place in our part of the country, and they may be springing up in yours if you look around for them. (We were once in New York City and ran across one there!)

At these markets you'll find a stunning array of the best and brightest of local seasonal produce plus such things as one-day-old eggs and home-cured olives, and, of course, plants and flowers. The price will almost always be less than, and the fruit and vegetables almost always twice as fresh as, in the supermarket.

Shopping in one of these open-air markets is also a joyful experience and a great stress reducer. The people (both buyers and sellers) are friendly and eager to tell you how to cook things you may not be familiar with and to offer new suggestions for the use of old vegetable friends. One Frenchwoman told us five new ways to prepare leeks while were lined up to buy them.

If you don't know if there are any markets in your area, try calling the local newspaper. That's where we've discovered most of those we go to. It's worth doing a lot of seeking to find something so life- and spirit-enhancing.

HEARTS AND FLOWERS

The dining atmosphere can be almost as important to your control as the diet. Mealtime should be a soothing respite from the stresses of the day.

Practicing what the Hindus call "one-pointedness"—concentrating on the enjoyment of the meal—is vital. A radio or TV shouting out the day's mayhem report is not conducive to mealtime tranquility. Neither are family arguments. A calm atmosphere helps you savor your food, and when you really taste what you're eating you can achieve a feeling of satisfaction with less food and thus will be less tempted to break your diet with a second helping.

Another way to leave the table not feeling hungry and yet not overeating is by eating more slowly. Although we don't advocate "Fletcherizing" your food—chewing each mouthful thirty-two times (once for each tooth), as was advocated by turn-of-the-century food faddist Harold Fletcher—we do feel it's a good idea to retreat from the frenzied chomp-and-gulp style of so many people in our hurry-up society. Aside from not really getting the maximum pleasure out of your meal, when you eat too fast your body doesn't have a chance to send your brain the "I am full" signal and you tend to eat more than you should or leave the table feeling hungry.

Another thing to remember is that candles and freshly cut flowers and other table enhancements contain no calories. Nor does it raise your blood sugar to arrange the food attractively on the plate. On the contrary, these very aspects of beauty at mealtime, along with a calm and loving atmosphere, tend to turn off the day's adrenalin and make control easier.

SOLO BITE

Joke. A man died and went to heaven. God greeted him and asked if there was anything he wanted. "As a matter of fact, yes," admitted the man. "I haven't eaten in a while and I *am* a little hungry."

"Fine, I'll go get dinner," said God.

While the man waited he passed the time by looking down below at the devil's domain, where the hellions were at their evening meal: beef Wellington, pheasant under glass, pâté de foie gras, the most luscious fresh fruits and vegetables, beautiful homemade rolls, fresh-churned butter, wine flowing like wine—everything anyone could want. The man was really salivating by the time God returned.

And what did God give him? A dry cheese sandwich and a glass of water.

"Gee, God," said the disappointed man. "I hate to complain, but how come they're eating all those terrific things down there and all you give me is a cheese sandwich?"

God sighed. "It didn't seem worthwhile cooking for just the two of us."

It's no joke that people living alone often feel it's not worthwhile cooking for just the one of them. Or if they do cook, it's as one friend of ours reported: "I knew I'd hit the gastronomic skids when I found myself standing by the stove eating dinner out of the frying pan."

Since 20 percent of America's households are now composed of one person and since many of these are older people who are into the years of high diabetes incidence, it stands to reason that there are a lot of people who are going to be tempted not to bother cooking "all that food" on the diabetic diet. This can cause real problems with their diabetes, especially since people in the maturity-onset category can often control their diabetes with diet alone if they follow the diet carefully.

June, who over the years of diabetes has often been a solo biter, always carefully presents herself with well-balanced meals based on the diet. For her this was a big general-health change for the better from her prediabetes days. Then she seldom planned meals in advance and would just drift vaguely toward the refrigerator and eat whatever she happened to find there. Not only does she prepare the diabetic diet now, but she treats herself the same way she'd treat a guest, presenting the meal as attractively as possible, pouring herself a glass of wine, listening to pleasant music, trying to make the meal a soothing, restoring experience in every way.

Change of Menu (formerly Menu Monthly) publishes two volumes of *Diabetic Cooking for One or Two,* each of which provides over 200 recipes (including exchanges) to make only one or two portions at a time. The Change of Menu Publications for diabetics are not generally available in bookstores, but you can order them directly from ads that appear in all the major diabetes publications and we always have them at the SugarFree Centers.

In a sense, diabetics living alone have an advantage in following the diabetic diet because they can have exactly what they should eat without feeling they're "imposing the diet" on hapless family members. Admittedly, though, it is more pleasant to dine with a companion (if he or she is a *pleasant* companion) than it is to dine alone. Loneliness can bring on depression, which can in turn cause you either to lose your appetite or to eat too much (or to eat things that are bad for you, like sweets) by way of compensation. And none of that is good for your diabetes.

If you live alone, why not get together with other solo biters and start a dining club to meet for dinner once or twice a week, taking turns fixing the meal or each bringing a dish? If you belong to a diabetes group maybe you could find a diabetic dining buddy and enjoy the challenge of fixing right-on-the-diet meals together. As Saint Paul said, "It takes two to keep the faith."

RESTAURANT ROULETTE

The greatest challenge to eating healthy meals comes as you cross the threshold of a restaurant. You have to read the menu as carefully as if you were trying to decipher a code (you are!), interrogate the waiter with the dedication of a member of the medieval Inquisition court, and turn the phrase "on the side" into a verbal tic that pops out as frequently as "you know" in some people's speech patterns.

The dangers you're trying to avoid in restaurants are too much sugar, too much fat—and just plain too much. Restaurants are as bad as commercial food processors when it comes to throwing in gratuitous sugar to "make food taste better." Indeed, sometimes they pose a double threat because they use commercially processed food to begin with and then compound the felony with their own wanton sugar spoon.

Although sugar can find its insidious way into anything, including vegetables and mashed potatoes, salad dressings and sauces are particularly risky. Even when you've grilled the waiter and he *swears* there's no sugar in something, you may not be safe. He may not know that a healthy (?!?) amount of sugar has been thrown in. We recommend *always* getting salad dressings and sauces on the side whenever possible, and if you're unsure about whether or not they're laced with sugar, we offer another suggestion from the ever-ingenious Dr. Dick Bernstein of the low-carbohydrate-diet fame: carry Tes-Tape or Diastix with you and discreetly dunk them into suspect substances. If they register below ½ percent glucose they're probably okay.

Here we want to insert a special word of caution about ordering soft drinks in restaurants. If your diet Coke, or whatever, does not arrive in a can or bottle, beware. One survey showed that about one-third of the time the diet drink was the real thing. Only Tes-Tape or Diastix will tell.

When it comes to fat, it's truly amazing how much a restaurant can serve up. Naturally, as a diabetic you'd never order deep-fried (or shallow-fried) anything, but restaurants like to throw fat on everything and often throw it on in a way that's difficult, if not impossible, to remove. Toast and English muffins come soaked in butter. Hot rolls frequently arrive with pats of butter melting over their brows. Vegetables swim in butter or, in the fancier restaurants, drown in hollandaise sauce. Meat suffocates beneath gravy; fish is buried in sauces. Never assume that *any* dish is going to arrive in a pure, unfatted state. On the side. On the side. On the side.

Incidentally, besides too much sugar and too much fat, restaurants generally give you (or, rather, charge you for) too much food, period. Both diabetics and nondiabetics who care about their weight and health need to have Great Dane–size doggie bags to carry out all the leftover food. Our solution is, whenever possible, to eat out at lunch rather than dinner. Or, if you're on a trip when you must eat all your meals out, try to eat the main meal at lunch and have the lighter meal (such as soup or salad and a sandwich) for dinner. This has several advantages. At lunchtime restaurants serve less food and charge less for it; the price of lunch in the best restaurants in town may be only around half what you'd pay for larger amounts of identical food at dinner. You can, therefore, enjoy haute cuisine and elegant ambience without breaking either your diet or your bank account. On top of that, if you eat your main meal at lunch you have a much better chance of walking or working off any excess sugar, fat, or calories you may have been unable to avoid.

Fast-Food-Chain Dining

Once, when we were musing on the idea that you can be taking excellent care of your diabetes but neglecting your health, the example occurred to us that you could follow the standard Exchange List diabetes diet while eating all your meals in fast-food chains. In that case, you would indeed be taking care of your disease but neglecting your health, because fast-food chains are very big on all those things you should avoid—sugar, white-flour products, salt, fat (most of it saturated or hydrogenated), and miscellaneous chemicals. They are also very small on those things you need for a healthy diet—fresh fruits and vegetables, fiber, whole grains.

But things are changing, thanks to health-conscious consumers. McDonald's has led the pack with its McLean Deluxe (91 percent fat free and 280 calories) and posted nutritional information and brochures on menu choices. Burger King is prominently displaying posters showing calorie content and the federal government's maximum daily intake of fat and sodium. This means the rest will soon have to follow suit to match the competition. So go to fast-food chains when it's convenient or when everybody else is going and you want to be part of the group. Just select the foods that are closest to your diet and don't make it a way of life.

CHAPTER 5
Exercise

When Barbara took a course in acupressure at Los Angeles Valley College a while back, it actually turned out to be a course in general health as well. (It was based on the book *Touch for Health Program* by chiropractor John F. Thie.) One of the main goals of the instructor was to get everyone in the class, whatever his or her age or physical condition, into an exercise program. By way of motivation she told a little story. It seems there was a guru who always gave the same advice when people came to consult him about their problems.

"I am sad," one would say.

"You ought to exercise more," was his response.

"I have no energy," another would say.

"You ought to exercise more."

"I can't sleep nights."

"You ought to exercise more."

We could play guru like this with all your diabetes-associated problems.

"I am overweight."

"You ought to exercise more."

"I am underweight."

"You ought to exercise more."

"I am always hungry."

"You ought to exercise more."

"My blood sugar is always high."

"You ought to exercise more."

"I keep having insulin reactions."

"You ought to exercise more."

"I am depressed and discouraged over my diabetes."

"You ought to exercise more."

"I want to get off the pills."

"You ought to exercise more."

"I have poor circulation."

"You ought to exercise more."

We could go on and on. No matter what ails you physically or emotionally, exercise helps. Strangely enough, it even helps contradictory conditions. Type II diabetics often have difficulty losing weight and juveniles sometimes can't gain. Exercise can help both problems.

SOLVING WEIGHTY PROBLEMS

It's not illogical that if you exercise more you will burn more calories and lose weight. But many maturity-onsetters argue that exercise just increases their appetites and that at best they stay the same weight and at worst they gain. Wrong. Studies done by nutritionist Jean Mayer have shown that vigorous exercise actually *suppresses* the appetite. When we were researching our book on biking (*Biking for Grownups*), we found that people on long bike tours had to be reminded that they should eat carbohydrate at regular intervals even if they didn't feel hungry. And they usually didn't feel hungry because of the body's failure to give the eating signal during sustained exercise.

Dr. Mayer made another interesting discovery. People who lose weight through exercise tend to be better at keeping it off than those who take if off through dieting. We read an explanation for this in *Fit or Fat* by physical-fitness expert Covert Bailey, who says a well-exercised body that doesn't have too much fat on it handles calories differently; it burns them at a high rate no matter what you're doing —even sitting still or sleeping!

We won't *guarantee* you'll lose weight with exercise. Something else may happen that's equally good. You'll lose fat, which will be replaced with muscle. Since muscle weighs more than fat your weight may remain the same but your measurements and appearance will improve vastly.

Your diabetes control is also likely to improve, because, as we mentioned earlier, overweight non–insulin-dependent diabetics often have *too much* insulin in their blood (hyperinsulinemia). The excess insulin is floating around along with excess sugar because obesity has made these persons' cells insulin-resistant, and the insulin can't unlock the cells and let the glucose in. The pancreas keeps getting high-blood-sugar signals and produces more and more insulin in a vain attempt to bring the blood sugar down. With exercise and a reduction of fat in the body, the cells become more receptive to insulin so that the sugar can get into the cells more easily and the pancreas can stop overproducing insulin. Therefore, you have the paradox of better control with less insulin. This is one of the reasons why overweight diabetics who reduce the fat stores in their bodies through exercise and proper diet can often get along without insulin or pills and, in fact, get rid of almost all their diabetes symptoms.

EXERCISING CONTROL

Exercise has special benefits for lean insulin-dependent diabetics, too. Those of you who have a regular program of sports activity have probably noticed that when you exercise you can put on needed weight and when you don't you tend to lose it. Why does exercise have the opposite effect than it has on overweight non–insulin-dependent diabetics? The answer is that with exercise the leans stay in better control and their food is totally utilized by the body instead of being thrown out and wasted as sugar in the urine. Also, when glucose from the diet cannot be adequately utilized, the body starts eating itself up, a kind of do-it-yourself cannibalism. Here's the experience of a diabetic physical-education professor we know: "I'm a rather lean, muscular 180 to 185 pounds. If I don't exercise I lose weight. My control is affected and my sugar levels increase. I then must return to my high activity level to gain it back."

Another benefit is that physically active insulin-dependent diabetics find they not only have less high blood sugar but less low blood sugar as well. In other words, exercise has a stabilizing effect on blood-sugar levels. The explanation of this is simple: (1) exercise helps glucose get into the cells (we like to think of it as a kind of "invisible insulin"), and thus helps reduce high blood sugar, and (2) it also helps the body build up its store of animal starch (glycogen) in the muscles and liver; this glycogen can be converted to glucose whenever needed, so active insulin takers have a good internal reserve of glucose for hypoglycemic emergencies and, hence, are less subject to low blood sugar.

EXER-HIGHS

Exercise simply makes you feel better all over—body and mind. This may be because for a while you're escaping from the pressure cooker of life as you exercise. And then again it may be the release of a hormone called norepinephrine. This hormone makes your spirits rise. A British medical team headed by Dr. Malcolm Carruthers found that only ten minutes of vigorous exercise was enough to double the body's level of this happy hormone and put a person in a better frame of mind.

Besides a rise in spirits, you get another kind of high from exericse. Dr. Ethan Sims and his wife, Dorothea, in their "Dialogue About Diabetes and Exercise" in the *ADA Forecast* for July/August 1974 quoted one of their friends describing his running experience.

> I also experience a type of "high" which has not often been commented on. The initial exhaustion of a run

> wears off in about five to ten minutes. About a half hour later, a gentle warmth begins to suffuse the lower limbs, which complements a state of complete physical relaxation. The sensorium is sharpened and thinking becomes more acute. A total sense of well-being which may last three to four hours permeates the event.

This high from exercise is for real. Diana Guthrie points out in her diabetes-education classes that exercise activates the body's endorphin system, and do you know what endorphin means? The morphine within. So you're getting yourself a perfectly delicious natural high with no harmful side effects. Well, maybe one. Just like the real stuff, the body's own morphine is addictive. Active sportspeople will tell you that when they have a day without their exercise fix they suffer withdrawal symptoms and become nervous and irritable.

But don't worry. Your addiction is what psychiatrist Dr. William Glasser calls a positive addiction, one that is good for you, one that makes you a stronger, healthier person in mind and body—and a better-controlled diabetic.

A MOVING MEDITATION

Another way that exercise makes you feel better is that, like meditation, it cleans your mind of the distressing mental debris—or it should if you're concentrating on your sport the way you ought to. If you're playing tennis, for example, and start thinking about the errands you're planning to do later or a fight you had with your spouse rather than about your game, you might as well walk off the court, because you're bound to lose. On the other hand, if your mind is totally on the tennis, you'll get a double benefit: your mind will be cleaned out and you'll have a much better chance to win.

The same is true of all sports. Downhill skiing is a particularly good example. Since it's such a basically unnatural sport—you have to lean out away from the hill when every fiber of your being wants to lean into it and cling—you have to really concentrate on what you're doing or SPLAT! You also need to be on the alert for hazards (human and otherwise) on the slopes. But another factor that makes skiing so great for ridding your mind of your troubles was summed up by a British businessman we once met in Lech, Austria. He said that skiing is the only sport he really likes. "When I'm up there on the slope," he said, "I forget about all of my business worries. I'm so bloody frightened that all I can think of is how I'm going to get down the hill in one piece." Skiing will even make you forget you have diabetes. Guaranteed.

FRIENDS INDEED

Exercise is also a great way to meet people. If you take up a sport, you soon acquire a new set of friends who share your enthusiasm. What's best about this for a diabetic is that your sports friends are the right kind of friends, the kind who will reinforce the healthy lifestyle you want to follow. They will be the kind who don't want to carouse around all night because they've got an early morning golf reservation or they're taking off at dawn to go hiking. If you meet someone in an aerobics class and decide to go to lunch together, it's not likely he or she will want to gulp down French fries and pecan pie with whipped cream: they've worked too hard to get in shape and won't want to blow it in a few moments of dietary indulgence.

Warning: There are some exercise fanatics who have what one psychologist termed "Yuppie Bulimia." These are people who spend half their time doing extremely strenuous exercise so they can spend the other half stuffing down food. Obviously, these are not the kind of friends you would seek out since they would be a bad influence on your diabetes in two ways.

YOU GOTTA HAVE HEART

At one American Diabetes Association meeting where we were carrying on about the virtues of exercise for diabetics, a gentleman in the audience asked if he really needed to exercise since his job involved physical labor. Probably yes. There are very few jobs that give you the right kind of exercise for optimum diabetes health. The only one we can think of offhand is that of the mail carrier who walks at top speed (a mile every fifteen minutes), rushing through the swift completion of those appointed rounds. And how many of them do that?

While all manner of exercise is better than doing nothing, the kind of exercise that produces the above-mentioned marvelous benefits for diabetics is aerobic exercise. Aerobic exercises are those that condition the heart, lungs, and blood vessels and lower cholesterol and triglyceride levels while increasing the body's ability to utilize oxygen. In other words, aerobic exercises ward off such cardiovascular problems as heart attack and stroke that plague the modern world in general and the diabetic population in particular.

Aerobic exercises are done:

1. **Continuously.** This means that the exercise must be done without stopping. If you're going to exercise for half an hour, you don't stop once during that entire half hour.
2. **Rhythmically.** A rhythmical exercise is one in which the muscles are contracting and relaxing on a rhythmical basis. Walking, jogging, running, hiking, cross-country skiing, swimming, bicycle riding, jumping rope, roller skating, rowing a boat—all these activities are rhythmical. You are moving yourself from one place to another under your own power in a steady manner. You can see that games like golf and tennis do not qualify—there is too much stop and go, which breaks up the rhythm.
3. **In intervals.** This word describes how you exercise continuously for your fifteen minutes, half hour, forty-five

minutes, or whatever. You work fast and then you alternate with an interval at a slower pace. Swim fast for two pool lengths, then slow for one; fast for two, slow for one—slow enough not to have to stop completely.

4. **Progressively.** This means that your exercise becomes progressively a little more difficult. When your body adjusts to one level of work load, you increase the amount you do. The trick is to progress in a lot of little steps.
5. **For endurance.** This word simply says that you're doing an endurance type of program, one that lasts more than five or ten minutes. Endurance activities improve your cardiovascular fitness, and that's the most important kind of fitness for a diabetic.

ACCESSIBLE AEROBICS

The following aerobics are readily accessible in that you can do them right out your front door—or even in the privacy of your home.

Running and Walking

As the Buddha said, "The only constant is change." Nothing has been more constant than our changing attitude toward running. When we wrote *The Diabetic's Sports and Exercise Book* we said, "Jogging and running bore the very sweatsuits off us." Then when it came to the original edition of this book we had become running enthusiasts—not fanatics the way a lot of runners are, but sweetly reasonable enthusiasts doing a mile to a mile-and-a-half almost every morning. This had come about partially as a result of what we learned when June was trying to cure her headaches. Dr. Otto Appenzeller in New Mexico discovered that running is an effective headache therapy. He also found that running creates the relaxation response not too unlike that attained by yoga, hypnosis, meditation, and the like—a toning down of the autonomic nervous system. And, as every dedicated runner will tell you, your whole life changes along with your body when you embark upon a rigorous running program. One study showed that runners are more likely to make major dietary changes for the better than participants in any other sport. Running also gives you a lot of exercise in a short period of time. It's true that you burn as many calories walking a mile as running a mile, but it generally takes longer. And time was the essence for us as it is for everyone these days. Running was also in style. Everyone was reading Jim Fixx's book and everywhere you looked people were stretching against trees and telephone poles and jogging and running and panting and sweating and training for marathons. As advocates of exercise, we could hardly not be runners.

Then styles changed. Jim Fixx's fatal heart attack while running dampened the enthusiasm a good bit. Actually, since he had a family history of heart trouble, his running probably gave him several extra years of life. Still, it provided a good excuse for people who wanted to stop running anyway. The medical reports also started coming in about the damage to knees and ankles from the incessant pounding, especially when the running was done on a hard surface, as it generally was, and especially for runners who were over forty as many were. Some Type A personalities (the intense, hard-driving, competitive sorts whom Dr. Meyer Friedman described in his book, *Type A Behavior and Your Health*) found that they were out running with a stopwatch, pushing for a faster time, a greater distance, putting greater pressure on themselves, just as they do on the job. Running, instead of reducing stress, was creating more.

We gradually climbed onto the new bandwagon of walking not running. Unless you have a passionate love for running, we suggest that you follow in our footsteps. Walking is the one sport that virtually anyone can do without risk. In fact, as one doctor put it, "It's impossible to walk too much." And the

Joslin Clinic unequivocally states in its manual, "Walking is the best exercise for your feet." We all know how important foot care is for a diabetic. And if you'd like a professional athlete's endorsement of walking, take Bill Talbert. On days when he doesn't play tennis, he makes it a point to walk forty to fifty blocks.

Here's the definitive endorsement of walking and other non-grueling physical activities. A study of 17,000 Harvard alumni revealed that you don't need to do arduous sports like running marathons to reap the life-saving benefits of exercise. Men who pursued such moderate activities as walking, climbing stairs, and sports that used 2,000 or more calories a week had death rates one-quarter to one-third lower than their more sedentary fellow-graduates. The life-saving benefits of exercise peaked at expending 3,500 calories a week. Burning more calories in exercise than that number in some cases proved to have a slight detrimental effect.

To determine how many calories you're burning in a particular activity so that you can reach the magic 2,000-a-week number, check the Chart of Calorie Expenditures in Appendix F.

One conclusion of the Harvard study was that a daily brisk three-mile walk will keep you fit and healthy and increase your life expectation.

You may even want to try racewalking. It really moves you along, and all the wiggling motion is a great reducer and toner. It's also enough of a recognized sport to be in the Olympics. One night a friend took Barbara out to a racewalking class. When they got there, there was a big crowd in the stands and a lot of people milling about. "Gee," mused Barbara, "I didn't know there was that much interest in racewalking. This sport is really catching on." It turned out that indeed there *wasn't* that much interest in racewalking. This was an all-comers track meet and racewalking was only a small part of it. About fifteen people were standing together in the racewalker corner. Two or three were experienced competitors; the rest, like Barbara and her friend, were there to learn and—unbeknownst to them at the time—to compete.

After about ten minutes of instruction, they were told that they would be walking a race. (That really chilled their marrow, but there was no way out.) Everybody lined up and then were off on a walk of four times around the track. In no time at all the experienced people lapped the learners and then lapped them again. After what seemed an interminable time, the only "competitors" left were Barbara and her friend. As the athletes were jogging and pacing around the periphery of the track getting ready for the 100 yard dash, a voice boomed over the loudspeaker, "The 100 yard dash is delayed. There are still two walkers on the track." That chagrin speeded them up a little, but it still seemed forever until they crossed the finish line. But as luck would have it, despite their dismal showing Barbara and her friend took a second and third in their age category.

Racewalking is easy to learn. After this brief and harrowing indoctrination, Barbara was able to teach June, and whenever not too many people are watching we break into the racewalk wiggle and it's truly a workout. If you're interested in trying it, look for a class—preferably one that doesn't involve a public competition at the end. Racewalkers are an extremely dedicated and evangelistic lot and they're delighted to sign on converts. If you can't find any classes or evangelists in your community, you could read *Racewalking for Fun and Fitness* by John Gray. (He tells you exactly how to do it and inspires you to action. Incidentally, although Gray is also a medal-winning runner, he considers walking the better sport.)

But whether you decide to go for running, jogging, racewalking, or just plain vigorous walking, as Dr. Joan Ullyot of the Institute for Health Research in San Francisco says, "the hardest step . . . is the first one out the door." If you're ready for this first step, this is how we suggest you go from there.

First, we suggest investing in a good pair of running or walking shoes. Fortunately, there are stores selling all kinds of these all over the country. Unfortunately, not all salespeople are knowledgeable about how to help you select the right kind of shoes and/or how to fit them correctly. Shop around and ask a lot of questions. One warning: please, we beg you, don't use tennis shoes for running or walking. They don't position your feet properly and are designed more for lateral than for forward motion. Also they don't protect you from the jars and jolts of the road, sidewalk, track, or ground. With the wrong shoes, these jars are transmitted throughout your body, creating trauma and stress.

Aside from the shoes, you can wear anything that's loose, comfortable, and appropriate to the weather.

Speaking of weather, don't let the weather provide you with an excuse. If you let the heat or the cold or the rain or the snow or the wind or the hail or the smog or the earthquake stop you, you'll wind up never running at all.

When should you run? We prefer mornings. Excuses seem to be easier to come by in the evenings, and if you run in the morning you can enjoy its benefits the whole day.

In June's running days, she ran before breakfast and immediately after her insulin injection. (After all, the old sports myth had it that you should never exercise after meals.) This worked pretty well until June started fine-tuning her diet and insulin therapy and began waking up in the morning with low blood sugar. She then found that after her run and after breakfast her blood sugar would go up into the 200 range. This baffled her until she remembered the Somogyi effect: hyperglycemia resulting from hypoglycemia—the body compensates for insulin shock by releasing too much sugar from its glycogen stores. Apparently she'd been running her already fairly low blood sugar into Somogyi territory. Sure enough, the first day she ran *after* breakfast, she found her blood sugar was only 110. Since then she has stuck to the "safe" time for insulin takers to exercise: after meals when the blood sugar is on the rise; it reaches its height one to one-and-a-half hours after a meal.

Before you go out you should always warm up with a few stretching exercises for the leg muscles—see the section of this chapter called "A Stretch in Time." As part of your warm-up routine it's also a good idea for the first few minutes of your outing to walk if you're a runner and to walk slowly if you're a walker. You should do the same thing for the last few minutes to cool down. And never take a hot bath or shower immediately after your exercise. You should wait for the blood to return to your innards from your feet and legs before you draw it away to the surface of your skin with hot water.

When you first begin your program, do it for only fifteen minutes. We prefer to work with time rather than distance. If you have a goal of a certain number of miles, you may try to run or walk faster to get them over with and get back to some project that's hanging over your head. This destroys the whole conditioning and relaxing aspects of the routine.

A good basic rule is to walk as fast as possible and run as slowly as possible. A slow run is at a "conversational pace." This means you're running slowly enough to carry on a conversation without getting out of breath.

And that's all there is to it. Keep at it every day (or with one or two days a week off), gradually increasing the total time and the amount of that time you spend running or walking. Your body will tell you when to make the increases: you may work up to a half hour or even an hour, and then again you may not. Don't stress yourself over it. Just do what feels right.

You may wonder what to do with your mind while you're doing all this with your body. Well, what you shouldn't do is stew over your problems and sort through all the things you should be doing instead of "wasting your time" exercising. That builds up the kind of stress that negates the benefits of the exercise. One thing you can do is combine meditation with your run or walk. Chant your mantra, count your exhalations, or do whatever best cleanses your mind of its incessant woe-churnings (see Chapter 8 on meditation). Or just look around and enjoy nature or people watching. You'll see a lot of things you miss when whizzing by in a car.

THE GREAT INDOORS

Although it's lovely to be out in the fresh air doing your exercise, sometimes the air isn't fresh. In Los Angeles we often have a smog alert and you're sternly advised not to go out to exercise in it. Or the air may be too fresh and freezing cold. Or in northern parts of the country in the winter there may not be enough daylight available to do your exercise if you're trying to fit it in before or after work. Or, especially if you're a woman exercising alone, you may feel a bit uneasy out walking or running by yourself in this hazardous world. Or it may be that you haven't quite worked your body into the kind of shape that you want to display on the city streets or country roads or athletic fields or tracks. In all of these cases, the answer may be indoor exercise. Here are a few possibilities.

Jumping Rope

This takes up very little space and takes almost no equipment (you can just use an old piece of clothesline). But if you want to get fancy, there are jump ropes available that rotate within the handles. You can get your heart rate up quickly with a vigorous period of rope jumping.

Aerobics

There are a lot of VCR tapes available for aerobics. They do a good job of keeping you motivated and moving and charting your heart rate so you don't overdo or underdo. There are also good TV aerobic programs. If you have a VCR, you can record them to use whenever it's convenient for you. In both of these cases, look for the "low impact" kind that don't do harm to your joints.

Rebounding

Doing aerobics on one of those rebounders or minitrampolines is an exhilarating exercise and, since the rebounder gives with each step, you can do the standard non–low-impact aerobics without joint problems. This is Barbara's favorite great indoors aerobic activity. The *Hooked on Aerobics* program from the University of Utah that appears on PBS is her favorite. The routines are entertaining, varied, and sound; and the people doing them are attractive but not extreme-bordering-on-weird in their appearance the way some aerobic performers are.

Exercycles

This is June's favorite. She works out every morning on an AirDyne so she can exercise her arms as well as her legs. Sometimes when she is reading or watching television or writing she rides a standard exercise bicycle so that she has her hands free.

Cross-Country Skiing Machines

These *really* give you a workout. It has been said that the cross-country skier is the world's most physically fit athlete. This includes cardiovascular fitness. These machines, however, do not come without some disadvantages: they're on the expensive side and take up a bit of space, both during use and in storage.

Rowing Machines

These are good for working out the upper as well as the lower body. They can often be tucked behind a sofa or bed so they don't intrude on your interior decor. There are even VCR tapes available that give you a rowing routine complete with peripheral outdoor scenery.

Tai-Chi

Tai-Chi is a system of exercise developed hundreds of years ago in China by Taoist monks, and it is still practiced by millions of Chinese people. The 108 basic moves use every part of the body. In Tai-Chi the body moves as one unit in a smooth, graceful pattern, almost like floating. Its basic principle is relaxation. Practiced twenty minutes a day, it builds up inner strength and has a tranquilizing effect.

Penny Foolish

In purchasing your exercise equipment, buy the best you can afford or maybe even a little better than you think you can afford. Ignore those super-bargain ads in the paper for brands of equipment you've never heard of. These are the kinds that are so unsatisfactory to use that they wind up hidden in a closet or gathering dust in the garage. Even if you stick to using them for a while, they often break down before you do. Especially beware of cheap exercycles and dinky little rebounders with feeble springs.

Women's Choice

In selecting a sport (indoor or outdoor), women should remember that unless part of your exercise is load-bearing, it doesn't help prevent osteoporosis, something we all want to avoid. Therefore, if your sport of choice is swimming, biking, exercycling, or rowing, remember to throw in some of the others that will get you on your feet and carrying yourself around. Variety is more fun anyway.

GOALS AND GUIDELINES

Gary Scherer, executive director of the Center for Heart and Health Improvement and director of Cardiac Rehabilitation at the Daniel Freeman Hospital in Inglewood, California, has come up with a very sensible exercise program for total health for everyone. With a few modifications it fits beautifully into a diabetic's exercise regime. He believes you should practice your exercise three times a week, or every other day. (We feel many young diabetics can and should exercise regularly every day.) The way the program goes is:

1. Fifteen minutes of stretching and flexibility exercises.
2. Five minutes of cardiovascular warm-up; moderate to brisk walking is ideal.
3. Thirty minutes of cardiovascular exercise—jogging, running, swimming, bicycling, jumping rope, aerobic or folk dancing, to name a few.
4. Five minutes of cardiovascular cool-down—reduced activity to allow the body to recover properly.
5. Enough sport and game activities to satisfy the competitive and social spirit.

The general guidelines for following your exercise program include:

1. Exercise regularly. The benefits of exercise cannot be stored; sporadic exercisers are subject to increased risks of injury.
2. Train, don't strain. Always exercise within your capacity. It is usually better to exercise longer than for brief periods at high intensity.
3. Time is in your favor. Take at least one month to get in shape for every year out of shape.
4. Exhale on effort. Breathe out during the effort cycle of muscular exercise (that portion of muscular exercise during the strenuous phase).
5. Avoid isometric exercise. It can significantly raise the blood pressure and place additional strain on the heart.
6. Don't exercise during illness. This may aggravate the problem, particularly with infectious diseases.
7. Never end with a sprint. The demands of a sprint after cardiovascular exercise may exceed the safe capacity of the heart.
8. Don't withhold drinking liquids. Adequate water

replacement during exercise is necessary to compensate for water loss through sweat and respiration.

9. Don't exercise through pain. If pain persists, call your personal physician.
10. Avoid extremes in temperature. Exercising in environments of extreme temperature or quick temperature changes after exercise, such as a very hot or cold shower or sauna, is dangerous.
11. Use sweat clothes properly. Sweat clothes are for warm-up, cool-down, and cold weather. Improper use can cause marked increases in body temperature, leading to heart palpitations or even death. Rubberized suits to promote heavy water loss are completely inadvisable.
12. Proper shoes. Weight-bearing exercises can place strain and trauma on the joints and muscles. Well-fitting and cushioned footwear can minimize or eliminate this. Proper choice of exercise surface can be beneficial.
13. No alcohol prior to exercise. Alcohol and many drugs constrict the vessels of the heart, and the increased demands for blood and oxygen during exercise cannot be met.
14. Reduce exercise level at altitude. The amount of oxygen available to your lungs and bloodstream is reduced and thus your exercise level must be reduced.
15. Avoid marked fatigue. It's not normal to be fatigued two hours after an exercise period.
16. Increase motivation. Participate in different physical activities; exercise with a group of friends; change locations.
17. Sweating is normal. Sweat is a normal by-product of metabolism of moderate to heavy exercise and helps cool the body.
18. Stop cigarette smoking. The harmful effects of smoking reduce heart and lung capacity.

Besides these general guidelines, we have a few special ones for diabetics.

Additional Guidelines for Diabetics Over Forty

Get a stress test. This will tell you how much exercise you can safely do. Barbara decided that since she's always telling others to get a stress test and since she's past the year of demarcation, she ought to take her own prescription. After getting wired up and trudging the treadmill, she was told by the doctor that "anything you *can* do won't hurt you." That is to say, if she *could* run the Boston Marathon or ski in the Vasaloppet or swim the English Channel she wouldn't get a heart attack if she did it.

Even if you don't intend to get into an active exercise program—although we can't imagine you wouldn't after the heavy hype we've given you—you should still get a stress test. Dr. George Sheehan, the famous proselytizer of running, says that a person who sits around doing nothing all the time is the one who needs a stress test the most because inactivity is one of the greatest stresses on the body.

Just to add the spice of medical controversy to the stress-test advice, the *New England Journal of Medicine* for August 2, 1979, reported a study which concluded that "the ability of stress testing to predict coronary-artery disease is limited in a heterogeneous population in which the prevalence of disease can be estimated through classification of the pain and sex of the patient." The news media immediately translated this as "those expensive tests are worthless."

June's doctor, an internist who specializes in cardiology and diabetes, translates it more moderately this way: "Essentially they are saying that the degree of accuracy [of the stress test] is directly proportional to the type of patient population that is being tested. They are also emphasizing that there is no substitute for an extremely accurate, complete history and physical examination. In summary, submaximal stress testing is useful only as a diagnostic adjunct to complete evaluation by a competent physician."

You might ask your own doctor for a translation.

Alternate your exercises. After forty it takes longer for your muscles to repair themselves after exercise, so it's best not to do the same exercise two days in a row—except, of course, walking, which you can't do too much of. For the more vigorous exercises, though, it's best, for example, to jog one day and ride your bike the next, swim one day and jump rope the next, or however you want to alternate.

If you're over fifty, it may be best to exercise only every other day. Again, though, this doesn't mean you should be inactive. You should keep moving, walking, climbing stairs instead of taking elevators, and being a generally vigorous person every day.

Do something. No excuses. Even if you're in your eighties or nineties, even if you have a heart problem, there are exercises you can do to improve the circulation in your feet and legs. These exercises act as an insurance policy against the dire things that can happen to diabetic toes, feet, and legs in advanced years. Figure 2 shows a series of exercises known as Buerger-Allen exercises. They should be performed before you get out of bed in the morning.

EXERCISE NO. 1

Lying flat on your back, lift your legs until they are perpendicular to your hips. From this position, with the soles of your feet facing the ceiling, move your feet up and down, bending them at the ankle, so that your toes are first pointing to the ceiling and then to the bed. Repeat ten to twelve times.

EXERCISE NO. 2

While in the same position, make clockwise circles with your feet ten to twelve times. Then make counterclockwise circles ten to twelve times.

EXERCISE NO. 3

Sit up and hang your legs over the edge of the bed, but don't touch the floor with your feet. Flex your ankles and point your toes first up, then down, as you did in Exercise 1. Do this ten to twelve times.

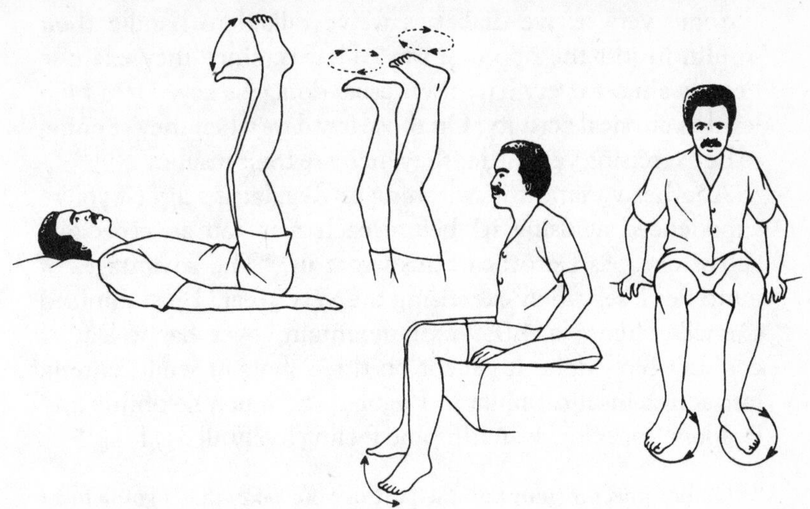

FIGURE 2
Buerger-Allen Exercises

EXERCISE NO. 4

Now, while in the same position, do the clockwise and counterclockwise circles you did in Exercise 2. Repeat ten to twelve times as before.

Additional Guidelines for Insulin Takers

When you exercise more than usual you must either take less insulin or eat more food. Diabetics handle this both ways, although there is a slight edge in favor of eating more because (1) a chance to eat more is always welcome to those on a restricted diet, (2) a lot of doctors don't want their patients to alter their insulin dosage, and, finally, (3) if you take your small hit of insulin in the morning and your big Exercise Event falls through for some reason or other, you're stuck with that low insulin dose all day and doomed to spilling or hardly eating.

Some very active diabetics we've talked to handle their insulin in just the opposite way. That is, since they exercise heavily almost every day, their usual dosage is keyed to a high level of physical activity. On those few days when they're going to be exercising very little, they increase their insulin.

Another variation is switching to Regular insulin (if you're experienced at using it) before each meal on an especially active day. As Dorothea Sims wrote us, "The advantages of multiple doses when exercising are very great. I just climbed Camel's Hump, a 4,089-foot mountain, over Labor Day. I couldn't have done it except on three shots of semi-Lente [a fast-acting insulin similar to Regular]. So much flexibility and freedom from clockwatching and feeling lively all day long!"

Do not inject insulin into the part of your body that's going to be active. Internists Veikko A. Kovisto and Philip Felig reported that insulin absorption is speeded up at the injection site if intense muscular activity is taking place there. This fast absorption could bring on a reaction. A bowler, therefore, should not inject the bowling arm before playing. A tennis player should avoid arms and legs on the day of a tournament. A skier uses the arms and legs all the time and—especially if a beginner—frequently the rear end as well, so the safest shooting spot on the day of a ski session would probably be the abdomen.

Do not exercise when your blood sugar is over 250 mg/dl. In this case, exercise can cause your blood sugar to go even higher.

Be prepared for lower-than-usual blood sugar for twenty-four hours after strenuous exercise. Exercise doesn't just lower your blood sugar during the exertion. There is a carryover effect in the evening, on into the middle of the night, and even the following day because exercise makes the body more sensitive to insulin action. Some diabetics report they have their more severe reactions on Monday after a sports-filled weekend. Be prepared.

ONE HEART BEATS IN THREE-QUARTER TIME

One way you can be sure you're getting enough of your aerobic exercise to strengthen your cardiovascular system, but not so much as to harm it, is to time your pulse. To find out the number of beats per minute, place two fingers on the inside of your wrist or three fingers on your neck on the side just below your jawbone. Using a watch with a sweep second hand, either count six seconds and multiply by 10, count ten seconds and multiply by 6, or count fifteen seconds and multiply by 4. For example, if you count twenty beats in fifteen seconds, your pulse rate is 80. Practice taking your pulse when you're not exercising until you can do it quickly and efficiently. You have to be fast and efficient enough to take your pulse when you *are* exercising without letting it drop while you fumble around trying to find it.

Gary Scherer recommends bringing your pulse up to 70 to 80 percent of your heart's capacity and keeping it at that level during your whole period of exercise (fifteen minutes minimum). Your heart's capacity is determined by your age and condition. Exercising at 70 percent capacity is for those of you who have any history of heart disease at all—and you should not do even that without a go-ahead from your doctor. If you're very out of shape, you shouldn't go over 75 percent; if you're young and in pretty good condition, aim for 80 percent of capacity. The 85 percent is *only* for an athlete in top shape and in training.

If you haven't done any exercising for a long time, you'll be amazed at how little it takes to get your pulse up to its 70 to 75 percent capacity. It may take only a brisk walking pace or even, in some cases, an average or slow pace. But don't be discouraged. If you keep at it, you'll find you're able to do more and more, faster and faster, with the same pulse rate and, voilà, you have good cardiovascular conditioning, a changed metabolism, better control, and another building block for your strong body.

A STRETCH IN TIME

In the list of guidelines for exercise and in our information on running there was the advice to do stretching before cardiovascular exercises. The ideal way to do this is with yoga. The benefits of yoga was another of the many life-change discoveries June made in her headache years. Yoga is the perfect companion to aerobic exercise—indeed, the perfect warm-up for aerobic exercise.

A diabetic of any age and in virtually any physical condition can benefit from yoga exercises. They are not jarring to the body and you are never supposed to strain yourself to achieve a position. Gradual, gentle, nonpainful stretching is the order of the day. Many people find it hard to believe that yoga exercises produce the wonderful effects they do, because they never leave you feeling exhausted and sore the way many people think exercises are supposed to.

We like yoga exercises for a dual set of reasons. First, they keep muscles and joints flexible, improve circulation, and free metabolism to work better. Second, they reduce mental as well as physical tension. They do this by making you slow down, because the positions are meant to be held for a certain number of counts rather than done in fast repetitions like some types of body-conditioning exercises. Also, yoga instructors (we should say hatha yoga, as that's the official term for the physical aspect of yoga) usually also teach deep-breathing techniques. Remember, we mentioned earlier in the book that fast, shallow breathing is a sign of body stress.

Now to get started with six special yoga positions especially helpful in preparing for aerobic exercises and for overall relaxation. These exercises will loosen all your muscle knots and keep you in condition for those more strenuous blood-sugar-lowering sports like jogging, swimming, bicycling, rowing, and hiking.

When doing these exercises try to develop a sense of body awareness. As yoga instructors advise, turn off your ordinary mind, the one that's forever churning like a washing machine, and really get into the stretch. Move slowly, smoothly into the stretch. *Be* the stretch. Experience it mentally as well as physically. As you breathe, feel you are actually breathing into the muscle you are stretching.

To do the exercises, choose a quiet room where you won't be disturbed. If the floor is carpeted, use a beach towel over it; on a hard surface, use a thin mat.

Abdominal Breathing (Figure 3)

Lie down on your back with your arms at your sides. Breathing through your nose, inhale, filling your abdomen with air—your abdomen, not your chest. To be sure, hold your hand on your stomach and make certain it balloons. Practice a few abdominal breaths until you know you're not chest breathing. Now inhale *slowly* through your nose to a count of four. Then exhale *slowly* to a count of six or eight, contracting your abdomen as you do. Repeat this slow, rhythmical breathing ten times.

Head Rolls (Figure 4)

These are sometimes called neck rolls, because the neck is the part of you that gets the workout.

Keeping your shoulders relaxed, simply drop your head forward with your chin close to your chest and then slowly roll your head in a complete circle, first to the left and then to the right. It's very important to roll slowly. A good technique is to pause several seconds when you get to your shoulder, pause

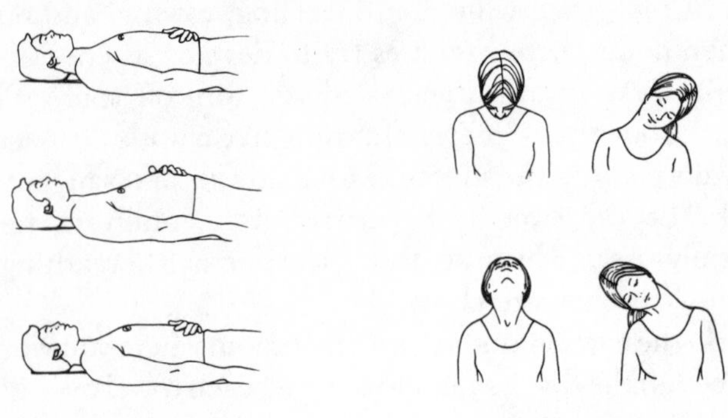

FIGURE 3
Abdominal Breathing

FIGURE 4
Yoga Head Rolls

again when your head is hanging backward, and again over your other shoulder. The more snap, crackle, and pop you hear when you do this exercise, the more you need the good it's doing you. When June first did head rolls, she heard a kind of pizzicato string-snapping quartet each time she rolled. Now that she's a regular yoga-exercise disciple she hears only an occasional bit of crackling.

After you loosen up, you should be able to do at least five head rolls. If they are too much for you at first, just drop your head forward and then drop it backward to stretch the throat. Hold several seconds in each position. Even this simple maneuver is very relaxing.

Chest Expansion (Figure 5)

Stand quietly for a minute with your arms hanging loosely at your sides. Bring them up to shoulder height, stretched out at your sides, bend them, and touch your fingertips under your chin.

Next, push your arms straight out in front of you and stretch your elbows. Now move your arms—still at shoulder level—around in back of you until you have to stop. Drop them and clasp your hands behind your back.

Keeping your arms as high behind you as you can, bend backward; drop your head back, too, as in a head roll. Hold for a few seconds.

Next, keeping your hands clasped behind you, bring your arms up over your head and bend at the waist until you've brought your arms as far forward as you can. Your head should now be hanging down near your knees. Your neck should be hanging loose. Hang that way for a count of about twenty. (Make sure your knees are not bent.)

Now straighten up slowly and you're ready for the second part of this exercise. Keep your hands locked together behind you. Put your left foot forward. Bend over until your forehead is as close to your left knee as possible without straining. To do this you have to bend your right knee. Feel those left-leg muscles stretch. Hold for a count of about ten.

Now straighten up and repeat with the right leg forward.

Do the entire routine—both parts of it—once more. There you are, revitalized and untensed.

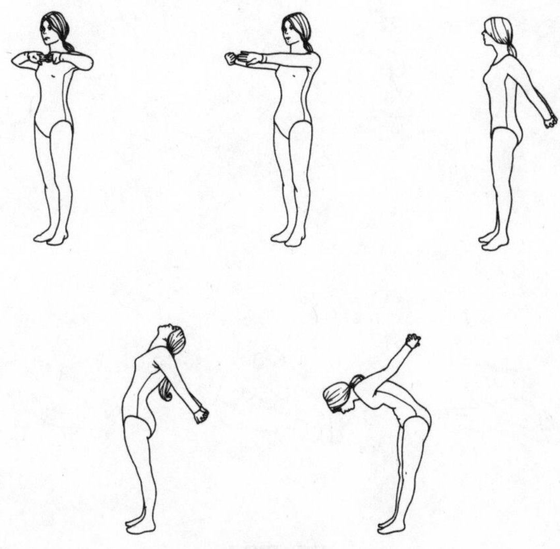

FIGURE 5
Chest Expansion

Alternate Leg Pulls (Figure 6)

Lower yourself to the floor and sit with your legs stretched out in front of you. Bend your right leg and, with your hands, bring your heel up close against the inside of your left, stretched-out leg.

Now raise both arms above your head, bend forward, and clasp your left leg as close to your ankle as you can without straining. Pull yourself down as far as you can. That may not be very far at all, but with time and practice you'll get your head down to rest on your knee. Be sure your neck is limp as you hold the position. After a slow count of thirty, let go and straighten up.

Do the same with your left leg bent and your right extended. Repeat the entire sequence twice.

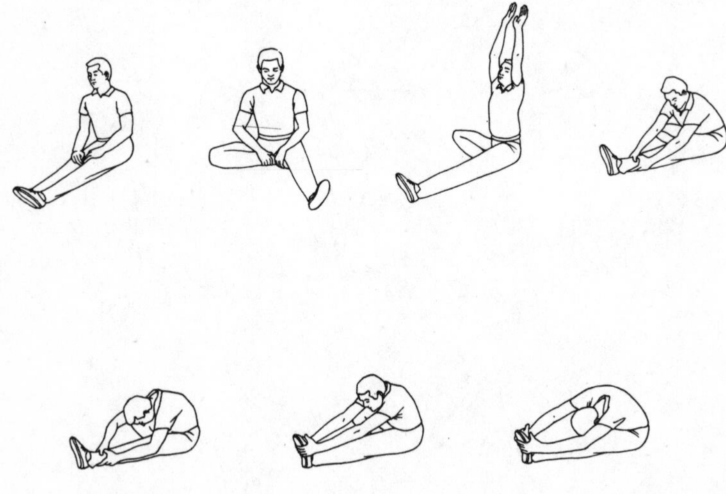

FIGURE 6
Alternate Leg Pulls

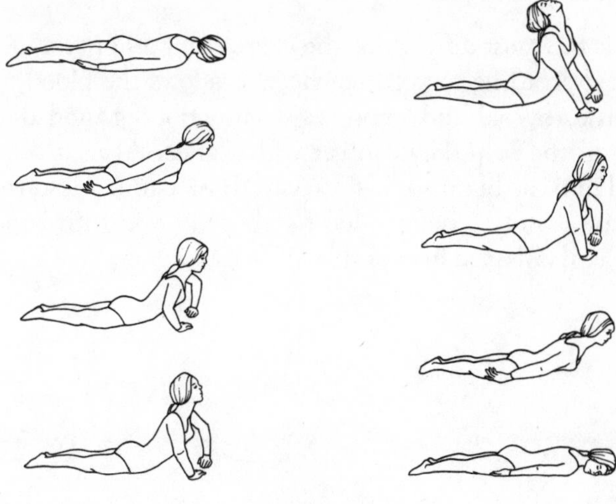

FIGURE 7
Cobra

The Cobra (Figure 7)

Lie flat on the floor face down with your forehead supporting your head and your arms at your sides. Go completely limp. Feel the tightness flow out of every muscle as you lie there playing dead.

Slowly raise your head and tilt it backward. Lift your upper body as far off the floor as you can without using your hands to help. When you're back as far as you can go without strain, bring your hands in under your shoulders, fingertips facing each other. Slowly push yourself up, your head tilted back toward your toes. Feel your spine arching. Keep your legs relaxed and your eyes closed. When you're back as far as you can go without strain, count to ten.

Lower yourself slowly. Bring your arms back to your sides as soon as you can and let your back muscles be in control as you lower yourself completely to the floor. Rest your cheek on the floor and go limp again.

Do the cobra twice.

The Plough (Figure 8)

This is the most difficult of the exercises, but it has a lot going for it. According to yoga teachers, it allows the blood to flow into the thyroid and improves its functioning, and diabetics need all the help they can get with glands. Also, it gets more blood into the brain so that you can think better. However, this exercise is not recommended for those of you with hypertension or an enlarged liver or spleen.

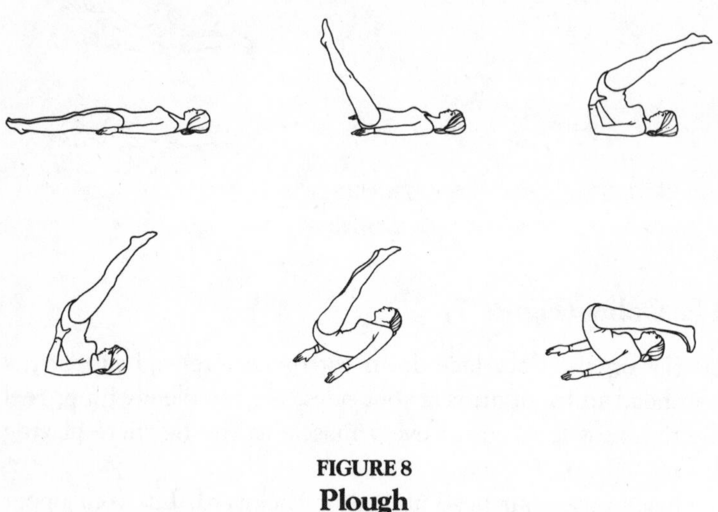

FIGURE 8
Plough

Lie down on your back. Place your hands along your sides, palms down. Slowly lift your legs, knees straight and together (the first times you do this you may need to bend your knees); and when they're high enough so that it's time to bend at the hips, move your hands up under your hips to brace yourself while you swing your legs into a vertical position. When you're in the correct position, your chin will be almost touching your chest. With your elbows on the floor and your hands bracing your hips, just remain "standing" on your shoulders for at least twenty seconds. (Those who do yoga regularly can hold this position as long as three minutes at a time.)

Now extend this shoulder stand into a plough position. Swing your legs backward with your toes pointing toward the floor. To brace yourself, put your arms on the floor with the palms of your hands down. Keeping your legs straight, lower your toes as far toward the floor as you can without straining or hurting. (Don't worry, you won't break your neck or back, nor will you topple over.) Stay in this position for the count of ten. Feel the stretch all along your spine. Roll out of the position and lower your legs to the floor without raising your head. The more you do this exercise the closer your toes will come to the floor, until they finally touch.

Relaxation Pose (Figure 9)

Lie on your back with your feet slightly apart, falling open naturally, and your arms at your sides with your palms up. Turn your attention to your cheek muscles and gently make sure they are relaxed. Imagine that a hand is gently stroking your hair and relaxing your scalp. Make a point of breathing through your nose and abdominally.

Lie in the relaxation pose at least three minutes. This is a good way to end your exercise session.

You may want to sign up for a yoga course at your local community college or recreation department. You can also check the program guide of the educational-television channel in your area to see if it carries either Richard Hittleman's *Yoga for Health* or *Lilias, Yoga and You.*

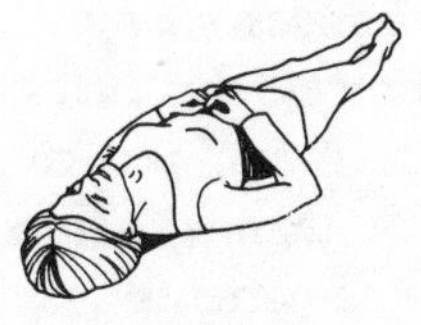

FIGURE 9
Relaxation Pose

MUSCLING IN

Just when we thought that with our regular aerobic exercise program we were doing the best we possibly could to promote a strong body, dissenting news started leaking out. The first thing that caught our collective eye was an article in *The New York Times Magazine* (April 26, 1991) entitled "The New Case for Woman Power." No, this wasn't a feminist exhortation for a female takeover of the world. The subject was weight training for women. Not only did it urge women to take up lifting weights because it "accentuates their natural curves, tightens the soft stuff of their thighs, stomach and upper arms and allows them to fit into smaller clothes," but it promised to help increase bone mass and thereby lower the risk of osteoporosis. Pretty compelling. Enough to start us thinking about going over to investigate a new gym that had just opened about a mile away.

Then, only a month later, there appeared an article in *U.S. News.* This one, called "Muscle Bound," loudly announced that "running, biking and other aerobic exercises are great for your heart, but they're not enough. To stay healthy, you've got to pump iron too." This is because 65 percent of the body's muscles are above the hips and most aerobic exercises do nothing to strengthen and develop them. Only "regular sessions of strength training can prevent and often reverse the progressive withering away of muscles. . . . Americans lose at least 30 to 40 percent of their strength and 10 to 12 percent of their muscle mass by the time they are 65."

Strength training does another great thing. When you convert fat to muscle it changes your metabolism so your body burns more calories, a process that helps solve weight problems. And, according to *U.S. News,* you can benefit from weight training at any age: "A team of Tufts University researchers . . . put nursing home patients ages 86 to 96 on a weight-training program designed to strengthen their legs. Although most of the men and women suffered from arthritis, heart disease, and high blood pressure . . . after only two months, the participants had doubled, tripled, and quadrupled their leg strength. Two patients developed enough leg strength to discard their canes."

The nondiabetic one among us was sold and ready to race over and join the gym, but the diabetic one still had misgivings. There have been reports over the years that weight training should *never* under any circumstances even be considered by a diabetic. They made it sound as if it would cause all the blood vessels in your eyes and kidneys to pop open and make your toes drop off.

We decided to do research among the more diabetically authoritative publications to see if strength training might actually be possible for diabetics after all, and might even have some special benefits for them. We found what we were looking for in the May/June 1990 issue of *Practical Diabetology:* "Weight Training and Diabetes Mellitus," by Richard M. Weil, M.Ed. He certainly had credentials enough to deliver an expert opinion: exercise physiologist in New York City, consultant to the Diabetes Treatment Center at the New York Eye and Ear Infirmary, and consultant to Park Avenue Diabetes Care.

The comment on the article by the editor had particular significance:

> A recent article in this publication recommended that people with diabetes not engage in resistance exercise (weight lifting). On publication of that article, I heard strong opinions to the contrary from a number of exercise physiologists. One of them, Richard Weil, was kind enough to put his thoughts into this excellent article, which has been reviewed by your editor, by a retinologist and by a physician well known for his research on diabetes and exercise.
>
> Many young men with diabetes enjoy weight lifting. Over the years, my colleagues and I have preached the party line and attempted to dissuade them from this form of exercise. To the best of my knowledge, we never succeeded in stopping anyone. Mr. Weil's article certainly

> provides us some reassurance. More important, it provides excellent logical guidelines so that our patients may participate safely in this form of exercise.

The article not only provided some reassurance, but lots of encouragement as well. Weil pointed out that the benefits of weight training for diabetics "include improvements in muscular strength and tone, glucose tolerance, body composition, muscle capillary density, osteoporosis, coordination, self-concept, and strength of tendons, ligaments, and joints." And he agreed with the *U.S. News* article, writing that the metabolism change brought about by weight training aids in weight loss.

He did emphasize that proliferative diabetic retinopathy would be the greatest risk factor in taking up weight training and that weight training should not be begun until the retinopathy has been stabilized with laser treatment and the ophthalmologist okays weight training. He also recommended evaluation and close monitoring by an ophthalmologist for those with chronic hypertension and/or moderate retinopathy.

For patients without contraindications, his conclusion was:

> Weight training can be a safe and potentially beneficial activity for virtually all patients with diabetes. Physicians should not overlook or dismiss this activity simply because they are unfamiliar with it or do not participate in it themselves. As primary providers of diabetes treatment, physicians should take the opportunity to inform interested patients about the potential benefits of weight lifting and encourage the development and maintenance of strength in patients of all ages.

That was green light enough for us. We marched right over and signed up at the gym and have been going at least three times a week ever since. We love it and have no intention of giving it up until we reach 100-plus.

Maybe you feel, as we did in the days before our enlightenment, that it's a waste of time to drive to a gym when you could get all the exercise you need at home or in the great outdoors instead of inside a damp and fetid building. In the first place, gyms are springing up everywhere, so you probably wouldn't have to drive very far to find one. In the second place, they aren't damp and fetid. The new gyms are clean and cool and well air-conditioned. (One caveat: if you're not a rock-music fan, don't forget to take your earplugs!)

And you definitely can't get all of this particular kind of exercise except by going to a gym—unless you build a complete gym in your home, as did diabetic diabetologist Richard K. Bernstein, M.D. For warm-up there are treadmills and exercycles and step machines. We prefer the exercycles, which, unlike the home variety, provide varying loads and speeds and take you up and down hills and on races and give you all kinds of other things to encourage you to work up a sweat. (Bring along a towel. It's gym courtesy to mop up your own sweat when you leave a machine.)

Then we move on to the Cybex machines. Our gym has both Nautilus and Cybex machines, as well as free weights. We always go for the Cybexes when they're not occupied because their cable system seems to work a lot more smoothly. (Free weights we're not interested in, figuring that we might drop one on a foot or strain a back by picking up one that's too heavy or using it the wrong way.) You adjust the machine to the proper height and to the weight you want to lift. For the latter, you just stick the weight pin into the number of pounds you're lifting. After you've been to the gym a few times this adjustment becomes almost automatic.

Then you progress methodically through machines that work the major muscle groups in your body. What we prefer—and recommend—is to start with eight to twelve repetitions (reps) using a weight we can lift on that particular machine without much effort. (We've heard it suggested that you start with 5 percent to 20 percent of your body weight, depending on what muscles you're using and what shape they're in.) In subsequent visits to the gym you gradually work up to twenty or thirty reps on that machine. (Psychological tip: counting backward as you work out—twenty–nineteen–eighteen, and so on—seems to make the time go faster than counting up in the conventional way.)

When you reach twenty or thirty reps, add another five or ten pounds, go back to eight to twelve reps, and work your way up again. Theoretically, in time, following this program, you'd get yourself up to thirty reps of one thousand pounds—in the way the hero of Greek myth Milo of Crotana lifted a calf shortly after its birth and, by lifting it every day, was ultimately able to lift a whole bull. Obviously it doesn't work this way, and you eventually reach a limit, although we feel we're far from that yet. Try not to be too macho about it—and this applies to women as well as men—grunting and groaning and straining to try to lift the heaviest thing you possibly can. For diabetics this is definitely a rotten idea, and we feel it's not such a hot idea for nondiabetics, either. While on the subject of women acting macho in the gym, we want to assure you that weight training won't make a woman *look* macho. To build up heavy bulky Schwarzeneggeresque muscles takes the male hormone testosterone. You know, that stuff that makes men want to do such things as start wars and cut in front of people in traffic.

To get the most benefit from your workout you shouldn't race through it. Take at least a couple of seconds to lift the weight, and double that to bring it back down. The consensus is that you breathe out on effort, although we've sometimes heard the opposite. One thing everyone agrees on, though, is that you shouldn't hold your breath, although there's a natural tendency to do so.

From warm-up to finish takes only about an hour for a good workout, and you emerge from the gym feeling strong and virtuous—because you are!

Although there are well-illustrated instructions on each machine, it's useful to have a trainer go around with you the first time or two. It makes it a lot easier and safer and builds up your confidence. In our gym one of the big selling points was that there were always trainers on the floor and you could even have one work with you every time you came in if you wanted to. This selling point turned out to be only that—a selling point. After our initial one hour of instruction, we hardly saw leotard or Avia shoe of the trainer again. We did track her down once to show us a new machine we couldn't figure out for ourselves.

This brings us to the business of gyms. We have noticed that the largest number of staff members of our gym are in the sales arena. Their job is to get the people to sign up and pay those initial charges. With ours there was an initial fee of $125 plus a "card fee" of $25. After that the monthly charge is $25. (This will vary depending on your gym.) From the battery of salespeople on hand (and the few number of trainers) we got the idea that the big thrust was to get as many people as possible to pay that initial sign-up fee rather than to be too concerned about how many people stuck it out for the long haul. If people never come back, that's fine because then there's room to sign up more. We chuckle and chortle over the fact that since we're not exactly Jane Fondas or Chers, when we signed up they were probably thinking, "Here's a quick fee. These two won't last a month." We fooled them!

What they do in our gym is only mildly scammy, just about what you'd expect in the modern world. We've heard of some gyms that were out-and-out frauds, getting hundreds of people to pay in advance for two or three years and then selling the gym to someone else who wouldn't—and wouldn't have to—honor the initial contract. So beware. Make sure the start-up fee isn't exorbitant, that they have a monthly fee rather than a contract for a year or more, that you can quit at any time with no penalty, and that if you're going to be out of town for a month or more, they'll waive the fee for that period.

Another piece of advice is to get a friend to sign up with you, especially if you, too, are no longer a teenybopper. It's a little intimidating to launch yourself alone into that sea of youth and beauty and muscle tone. It will also keep you going regularly. Invariably on the day one of you isn't in the mood to go, the other will be and will drag you along.

So our advice is for you to add weight training two or three days a week to your exercise program. Make it a part of the weave of your life, as a weight-training enthusiast friend put it.

Of course, you should check with your doctor before embarking upon such a program. If he or she says no, ask if there's a specific reason. (For example, "You have proliferative diabetic retinopathy.") If the response is just something like, "Weight training is not a good idea for diabetics," you should refer him or her to the *Practical Diabetology* article. You could even order a copy of that issue of the publication yourself and have it at the ready in case you get a negative response without justification. (*Practical Diabetology,* 150 West 22nd Street, New York, NY 10011. Request Volume 9, Number 3, May/June 1990. It costs $8.00 plus $2.50 shipping and handling.)

Keep in mind that it wasn't too many years ago that diabetics were forbidden by their doctors to take part in *any* exercise, and today exercise is recognized as a cornerstone of diabetes control.

PART II
A Tranquil Mind

Now that you've become aware that reducing physical stress through a healthful diet and exercise can also calm your mind, we want to show you how reducing mental and emotional stress will help create a tension-free body.

This intimate connection between mind and body, long recognized by Eastern societies but neglected in the West, is finally coming to the fore in America. Researchers at the Menninger Foundation have proven scientifically that every change in the body produces a change in the mind, and every change in the mind produces a change in the body.

As a diabetic you may have had considerable experience with the body-mind/mind-body effect. Say, for example, you don't have time to eat your usual quota of breakfast and in midmorning your blood-sugar level drops below 80, into hypoglycemic territory. Now, this is a purely physical happening, but what does it do to your *mental* processes? We don't really have to tell you but, just for review, you get irritable and hostile, confused and indecisive—you "go goofy." Such is the power of the body over the mind. As Kurt Vonnegut has as the continuing theme of his *Breakfast of Champions* when someone does something outrageous, "his chemicals made him do it."

On the flip side of the body-mind coin we have for an example a recent event in June's life. It was during the period when she was conducting the high-carbohydrate, high-fiber-diet experiment on herself. Barbara phoned her just before dinnertime and announced, "Guess what? Because of Proposition 13 the college district office has decided we librarians are to keep the library open during Easter vacation week with no extra pay, as voluntary work overload." June hit the ceiling like a French champagne cork. That evening when she took her blood sugar one hour after dinner it was well above 200. At first she couldn't explain this sudden failure of the diet, because she'd been having normal blood sugars for more than a week. Was it too large a potato, the unmeasured popcorn before dinner, extra-sweet strawberries? No. The truth finally struck home. It was her mental rage, the emotion directed against an unfair and arbitrary ruling. And sure enough, after an almost identical dinner the next evening all was well in blood-sugar land, because all was calm in her mind.

BIOFEEDBACK

Biofeedback is the most palatable of the new unstressing techniques to the skeptical scientists. They can't deny the mind-body connection when they see it proved on a machine. The way biofeedback works is that you are hooked up to electronic instruments that feed back to you information about what is happening inside your body (your temperature, your pulse, your muscle tension, the speed of your brain waves). Using this information, you learn to control these internal body processes.

Because biofeedback training has been successful in helping people reduce symptoms in a number of stress-related diseases, such as high blood pressure and headaches, two investigators—Thomas H. Budzynaki and Richard L. VandenBergh of the University of Colorado Medical Center—tried biofeedback-relaxation training with a twenty-year-old diabetic student who had been in the hospital eleven times with ketoacidosis (acid poisoning) during her first year in college. The doctors thought emotional upsets had contributed to her loss of diabetes control. Not only did learning "cultivated relaxation" help her lower her daily insulin from eighty-five units to forty-three, but she had no more hospitalizations for ketoacidosis and she felt that the technique helped her control her anxiety and tension levels and thereby stabilize her diabetes.

DIABETICS' CHOICE

A few of the more advanced diabetes-education centers, such as the Diabetes Treatment Center in Wichita, Kansas, are offering instruction in the newer methods of reducing physical and mental tension. Diana Guthrie, who works with her husband, Dr. Richard Guthrie, in the Kansas Center, teaches several different stress-reducing techniques in her classes for diabetics and their family members and friends. She not only explains biofeedback to her students but gives them a practice exercise with a thermometer to show them how they can raise the temperature of their hands through the power of the mind. (Warm hands usually mean you are relaxed; cold hands mean you are tense.) She also gives her students a sampling of other techniques, such as deep-muscle relaxation (progressive relaxation), meditation, and guided imagery. She advises them to practice any of these methods that appeal to them for five, ten, or fifteen minutes a day for better control of their diabetes.

We're going to give you instruction in four different unstressing techniques: progressive relaxation, autogenics (self-hypnosis), meditation, and guided imagery. Only you can choose which ones seem to be right for you; there is no proven difference in their effectiveness. The best results, however, are obtained by combining two or more of these therapies.

A final tip is that you get results from these therapies only if you adopt a let-it-happen attitude. Paradoxically, the less you try, the more you progress. How do you manage to soft-sell these therapies to yourself? The directions we've read include such admonitions as "have a creatively expectant attitude" and "plant the seed and let it grow." But perhaps the most graphic and understandable description we've come across is the one that compares the method of performing these techniques to urination: "Just relax and let go."

CHAPTER 6
Progressive Relaxation

Exercise therapists say that one of their greatest challenges is just getting people to know what a relaxed muscle feels like. Many of us have been so tense for so long that we consider muscular tension to be our natural state. These exercises are for those of you who can't tell a tense muscle from a relaxed one.

Progressive relaxation, or deep-muscle relaxation, as it's sometimes called, is a system of first tensing a part of the body and then untensing it in order to feel the difference and thereby become capable of making the transition from tension to relaxation yourself. It was developed over fifty years ago by a Chicago physician, Edmond Jacobson.

Dr. Jacobson based his method on laboratory experiments which proved that when your muscles are completely relaxed so are your mind and your emotions. And what are relaxed muscles? They are muscles that are totally limp—that is, you are neither contracting (tightening) them nor holding them rigid.

Progressive relaxation is a very easy technique to learn, but it does require patience. It takes most people two or three weeks to learn the techniques if they practice half an hour a day, five days a week. You can hire a therapist who specializes in "Jacobsonian therapy," you can buy mail-order tapes to use at home, or you can learn to do it yourself by reading our directions here.

The training program depends on (1) repetition—that is, *daily* practice—and (2) effortlessness, because the less conscious effort you bring to untensing the muscles, the more relaxation you attain. It's the old art dictum of "less is more."

Over and over in the learning sessions you experience the difference of sensation between extremely tense and extremely relaxed muscles until you can recognize the difference without any doubt or hesitation. Once you know exactly what your muscles are doing, you'll not only be able to control your tendency to tense up but you'll become aware when you're locking some part of yourself into a stiff, awkward posture that will eventually become your "natural position." In this way you'll be able to avoid developing chronic tension in that set of muscles.

Now let's go through a practice session of progressive relaxation. You may want to have someone read this to you at first or, if you have a tape recorder, you may prefer to record it and listen to yourself telling yourself what to do. The value of this entire procedure is to plunge you into tension and then have the tension dissolve as you let go. You really only have to *think* about tightening a body part to engage the muscles, but in this practice session we're exaggerating to illustrate the contrast between tight and loose. Work slowly, holding each tension position for twenty to thirty seconds.

Sit in a high-backed chair or lie on your back on a carpeted floor or mat. Take a deep breath and hold it a moment. Breathe through your nostrils and from the abdomen, if you can. As you exhale slowly, try to let go of tension. Keep up a rhythmical pattern of breathing for a couple of minutes.

Direct your attention to your right hand. (If you are left-handed, start with your left hand and revise the following instructions accordingly.) Clench your fist tightly. Observe your forearm; see it become tight, too. Hold. Stretch your fingers out and allow yourself to relax again after twenty or thirty seconds of tension. Be aware of what is happening to your muscles, but don't be judgmental.

Make another tight fist with your right hand. Be aware of your muscles all the way up to your elbow. Hold. Let go slowly. Sense the difference between tenseness and relaxation.

Now, direct your attention to your left hand and make a tight fist. Notice how your arm feels. Hold. Slowly let go.

Next, push down on your chair or the floor with your right hand. Sense how your upper arm tightens. Hold. Relax and feel the flow of energy leaving. Now push with your left hand, hold, and then let go.

Hunch your shoulders so that you feel tension in your shoulders and in the back of your neck. Make it extreme. Hold. Then float down. Let your shoulders fall. Sense the muscles tense and then feel them relax.

With your hands, arms, and shoulders relaxed, push the back of your head hard against the chair or the floor. Sense the tension in the back of the neck. Hold. Then relax and let your head float.

Now the chin. Tighten it. Clench your teeth. Hold. Then relax and allow your mouth to open a bit. Be slack-jawed.

Push your tongue against the roof of your mouth. Hard. Hold. Then allow it to flop down. Notice how it seems to get larger as it relaxes.

Tighten your eyes. The "purse-string" muscles go around them. Close the purse. Hold. Allow your eyes to relax slowly.

Frown. Make a deep above-the-nose crease. Slowly relax. Do this particular exercise three times.

Next, raise your eyebrows all the way up. Hold until you get the feel, then lower.

The scalp muscle runs from the edge of the hair line to the back of the head. If you push your eyebrows, your ears, and the back of your head upward, you'll be contracting your scalp muscles. Hold. Now let down.

Tighten the muscles below your shoulders by arching your back. Hold. Then relax.

Next, tighten the abdomen—make it hard. Hold, and slowly let go.

The final step is to tighten your legs and feet. Stiffen your right leg. Hold. Relax it. Make your left leg rigid, hold, and then let the muscles smooth out. Study the feel of long, stretched-out, expanded leg muscles. Curl the toes of your right foot, making a "fist" of your foot. Hold. Then let go. Do the same with the left foot. Tighten, hold, release.

You will feel totally released from all tension—muscular or otherwise—at the end of your progressive-relaxation practice session. You will feel good all over. The more you practice, the deeper your relaxation.

As you gain skill you can streamline your sessions and relax without tensing first. Just quickly check the different muscles in your mind.

The final stage of deep-muscle relaxation is to relax all of your body at the same time. Check for feedback from different muscles and relax any that feel tense. Finally, you should be able to relax all over in only twenty seconds or, if you get to be championship caliber, in only five seconds. Jacobson's goal with his patients was to teach them to relax muscles as quickly as they could contract them.

CHAPTER 7

Autogenic Training

Autogenics—the word means "self-generating"—is a tension-relieving method that involves repeating short self-hypnotic sentences to yourself in order to influence your body to relax. For example, "My right arm is very heavy" is the first suggestion you give your body to help your muscles relax. You concentrate on creating, first, feelings of heaviness and then feelings of warmth. Feelings of heaviness indicate relaxed muscles and feelings of warmth indicate that blood vessels have dilated (relaxed). Once your right arm is heavy and warm, the body communicates this message to other muscles and you slip into a generalized total-body state of relaxation.

Autogenic training was perfected in Europe in the 1930s by a German doctor, J. H. Shultz, and has been widely known and used as a therapy there, but it is only now catching on in the United States. In Europe the training is usually given by physicians. Americans are being introduced to it through pain clinics and self-help books.

We're going to teach you the autogenic training formulas in stages, because that's the best way to learn them—in fact, the only way to learn them. We'll divide Dr. Shultz's original script into six parts: (1) heavy arms and legs, (2) warm arms and legs, (3) calm heartbeat, (4) regular breathing, (5) warm abdomen, and (6) cool forehead.

We recorded a cassette tape of the entire autogenic-relaxation script as presented here and used it ourselves over a period of several weeks, and also tried the tape on several friends. We found that it works well for almost every accepting person whose mind is not closed to self-hypnosis.

In the beginning you are supposed to practice three times a day—after lunch and dinner and before going to bed. You can either lie down on a couch or bed with a pillow under your head and neck, assuming the yoga relaxation position, or sit in a high-backed straight chair.

Close your eyes, breathe deeply, and exhale slowly a few times to get general body relaxation, and then *slowly* repeat to yourself the following sentences. As you say each sentence, concentrate on that part of your body and feel it doing what you are telling it to do.

STAGE 1: HEAVINESS

My right arm is heavy. (*Repeat each sentence four times.*)
My left arm is heavy.
Both arms are heavy.
My right leg is heavy.
My left leg is heavy.
Both legs are heavy.

STAGE 2: WARMTH

My right arm is warm. (*Repeat four times.*)
My left arm is warm.
Both arms are warm.
My right leg is warm.
My left leg is warm.
Both legs are warm.

STAGE 3: CALM HEARTBEAT

My heartbeat is calm and regular. (*Repeat four times.*)

STAGE 4: REGULAR BREATHING

My body breathes itself. (*Repeat four times.*)

STAGE 5: WARM ABDOMEN

My abdomen is warm. (*Repeat four times.*)

STAGE 6: COOL FOREHEAD

My forehead is cool. (*Repeat four times.*)

At the end of your practice sessions you have to bring yourself back to an active state, canceling or inactivating the training formulas by saying, "Arms firm, breathe deeply, open eyes." You have to be very careful not to forget this canceling sentence or you'll be trying to go about your regular activities with various parts of your body semi-hypnotized.

It may take you no time at all—only a session or two—to get through stages 1 and 2 and warm your arms and legs. And then again it may take you several weeks. We have to be so vague because it all depends on how suggestible you are. Some people, Barbara among them, have only to let a thought walk once across their minds and their bodies pick it up and go into action. Not surprisingly, therefore, it took Barbara only one session of autogenics to be able to warm her hands to the point of practically being able to fry eggs on them. June's suggestibility was initially much lower, but with practice she's increased her mind power amazingly.

Spend as much time as you need to on each stage in order to master it completely before going on and adding the next one. When you can go through the entire sequence of formulas from heavy arms to cool forehead in under five minutes, you can abbreviate the sequence into "My arms and legs are heavy and warm...heartbeat calm and regular...my body breathes itself...my abdomen is warm...my forehead is cool..." plus the canceling formula, "Arms firm, breathe deeply, open eyes."

When you advance to this point you can add additional autosuggestions directed specifically at helping you control diabetes or diabetes-related symptoms. Dr. Hannes Lindemann, author of *Relieve Tension the Autogenic Way*, suggests that a diabetic might say, "Pancreas flowingly warm," but we find that sentence not flowingly smooth (it's a translation from the German). Maybe you'd prefer some suggestion of your own devising, such as "Pancreas working calmly and perfectly" or "My blood sugar is normal."

We'd like to warn you not to get discouraged if you experience the slipping-back syndrome. That is, you may seem to deteriorate in your ability to respond to these self-commands, but with continued practice you will surge ahead again. Also, there is the possibility of what are known as "autogenic discharges" during the practice sessions. These are such things as muscle twitching, trembling, crying spells, and nausea. They're perfectly normal when unstressing, and meditators experience them, too. Just don't feel frightened if they should happen to you.

What we ourselves particularly like about the training is the total body relaxation we can achieve with it. In fact, we both still use autogenic formulas for putting ourselves to sleep at night after a tension-filled day. June uses them for putting herself back to sleep if she wakes up in the wee hours with a reaction and has to get up and eat a snack.

CHAPTER 8
Meditation

Meditation comes out of Eastern mystical tradition. We're concerned here not with the the complex, centuries-old religious teachings of Buddhism associated with meditation, but with meditation as a relaxation and calming technique. It's our impression that some doctors shy away from recommending it because of its religious implications. But to quote Eknath Easwaran, author of *The Mantram Handbook,* "Meditation is not a religion; it is a technique which enables us to realize for ourselves the unity of life within any of the world's great religious traditions, or even if we profess no religion at all."

Meditation is a generalized unstressing technique that releases you from your thinking machine, from that restless voice inside your head that never lets up on you except when you're asleep or unconscious. What we particularly like about meditation is that if you carry it off, it gives you a wonderful respite from that problem you carry around in your thoughts all your waking hours—your diabetes. If you practice consistently, meditation can change not just your physiology but your entire life.

BUSY DOING NOTHING

The objective in all meditation is to control the attention. What you do is block out the outer world and submerge yourself in your own inner world. Each school of Buddhism, each branch of each school, even each yoga or Zen master seems to have a particular set of instructions for how to do this. Transcendental Meditation (TM) is the meditative technique most of us have heard about, because it's been well publicized and advertised in the United States by its founder, Maharishi Mahesh Yogi. In TM you restrict your attention by repeating a sound (mantra) over and over again while sitting with your eyes closed. TM is based on an East Indian form of Buddhism. In Zen, the Japanese form of Buddhism, you open up your attention by concentrating on your breathing.

We're going to discuss here only the beginning exercises for each of these two types of meditation. What we tell you may sound simplistic, but, believe us, only the explanation is simplistic. The process itself is extremely elusive and takes dedication to master. Until you've tried it, you can't realize how almost utterly impossible it is to harness your mind or turn it off for even a few seconds, let alone for half an hour. (You *can* do it, however.) Nor can you realize what a stunning relief it is from your normal state of awareness when you finally manage to do it, even briefly.

WHERE AND WHEN TO MEDITATE

Meditation should always be practiced in the same place, someplace where you will not be interrupted and where there is no noise. Finding this serene atmosphere is often the biggest challenge. June uses a small dining room that looks out onto the patio.

There are numerous traditional positions for meditation. Full lotus (Figure 10) is the classic, but half lotus (Figure 11) and sitting on the edge of a chair (Figure 12) are perfectly acceptable for beginners and those who don't want to cut off so much circulation. Select the one that suits you best.

June finds it a good practice to meditate at the same time each day, and looks forward to this time as free from stress.

Early morning on arising and before taking her insulin is the best time for her. (Meditating after eating is not recommended.) Before dinner is good, too, but before going to bed is not, as it may heighten your consciousness so much that you can't get to sleep.

Start with five minutes a day and gradually extend the time until you can handle as much as half an hour. A short meditation done daily is far preferable to a longer one done erratically. And if you have to change time or place occasionally, do so rather than eliminating that day's practice entirely. You need regular practice to create that oasis in your daily life where stress dare not visit you.

TRANSCENDENTAL MEDITATION

Let's begin with transcendental—mantra or sound—meditation and then go on to Zen—breathing—meditation. The first step is to choose your sound. The mantra is usually short, as short as a single syllable or two, and should have a melodious sound. The TM'ers say it should have no special significance, but in much Hindu yoga practice the mantra is often an inspirational passage of several syllables or even words. Patricia Carrington, a Princeton University psychologist who uses meditation for mental therapy in her counseling practice, suggests that students in her program pick whichever of the following mantras sounds to them most pleasant and soothing: Ah-nam, Shi-rim, or Ra-mah.

We ourselves like Diana Guthrie's idea of choosing a scripture to meditate upon. She uses "Be still, and know that I am God" (Psalms 46:10). Each time, as she repeats this verse she makes it a shorter and shorter mantra by gradually eliminating words until she is down to the two words "Be still" and finally just "Be."

To do your mantra meditation, go to your chosen spot and take your chosen position. Take a few slow, deep breaths to quiet yourself, but not so deep that you become light-headed.

Then close your eyes and start repeating your mantra slowly to yourself over and over again, breathing abdominally through your nose. As extraneous thoughts and images crowd into your mind, just let them flow through without allowing them to distract you from concentrating on your mantra. (When you are in this state, you cannot concentrate on any aspect of your diabetes.)

When you meditate it is something like placing yourself in an isolation chamber. And like the other unstressing techniques, it's virtually an impossibility to explain how to do it. In fact, some Indian teachers say that you don't "do" it. You create in yourself a state of nondoing and meditation happens spontaneously.

When you finish, stop repeating the mantra and sit, with your eyes still closed, for several more minutes. Rather than snapping yourself out of your meditative state, open your eyes, stretch the way you would when awakening from a nap, and then get up and resume your normal activities. You will feel refreshed and energized.

ZEN MEDITATION

Turning now to the Zen technique, how you sit is very important. Use the full- or half-lotus position, or sit on the forward part of a straight chair. Your spine should be straight and the small of your back concave (abdomen pushed out) and your chin pulled in. Keep your hands in your lap, turned up, with the left hand inside the right, unless you're left-handed; in that case, the right hand should be inside the left. Your thumbs should be lightly touching. Keep your eyes open, looking about three feet in front of you and downward, but unfocused. Begin by moving your torso in a wide circle, gradually narrowing the circle until you come to a stop at your natural center, where you will feel balanced and secure.

Now sit there and let your mind follow the movement of your breathing. Use abdominal breathing: in and out, in and out.

Let other thoughts and images come but also let them go as you continue concentrating on your breathing. You can count one as you exhale if this helps, or one as you inhale and two as you exhale. You can even count your breathing all the way to ten, but no higher, as it would be distracting. Eventually you will get to the point where you can just sit and feel your breathing without counting. In fact, Zen teachers (roshis) refer to Zen practice as "just sitting."

MEDI-TEACHERS

Many meditators feel that for any form of meditation you should work under the direction of a teacher, because you need someone to answer your questions and help you with uncomfortable emotional and physical side effects that may appear as you are becoming unstressed, the same as with autogenics. Our suggestion for finding a teacher is to check with community and four-year colleges in your vicinity. Many offer courses in meditation, and the classes are sometimes held at the headquarters of yoga or Zen training centers. Meditation sessions with a Christian emphasis are offered by some churches. You can find announcements about these in your local newspaper.

CHAPTER 9
Guided Imagery

Guided imagery, or visualization, as some therapists call it, is the act of forming images in your mind to calm yourself or to solve life's problems. This technique offers you two important benefits. First, it allows you to escape from your daily tensions into a tranquil haven; second, once there, through the eyes of an imaginary advisor you are at last able to look at the big picture of the whole integrated mind-body-environment complex of your life and see what out-of-focus elements are responsible for increasing your tensions and/or causing your blood sugar to bounce around.

As a technique of self-therapy, guided imagery has very respected credentials among therapists and psychologists, and recent studies of the brain's hemispheres are helping scientists understand how guided imagery works.

The brain has two hemispheres. The left hemisphere controls the right side of the body; the right hemisphere controls the left side. The left hemisphere is the verbal, logical half. The right hemisphere is where your intuition and creativity abide. This side works not with words, but with pictures, with images. For calming yourself and solving your problems, one guided-imagery picture from the right hemisphere is worth a thousand words from the left.

As the name of the technique suggests, you need a guide to lead you out of your left hemisphere and into your right. Diana

Guthrie is such an experienced guide for diabetics that we're going to let her take you on your first guided-imagery journey the way she does in her classes.

> Get really comfortable. If you have something tight on, loosen it up. Close your eyes, because this is something between you and yourself. Now listen to my voice. Think through what I am saying.
>
> First you see yourself inside a box. It looks as if there isn't any way for you to get out of the box. You feel very crunched, very enclosed. This box can sometimes represent your diabetes or your problems or your fears. You look up and you see a hand reaching down for you. That hand could be a family member or a friend or your heavenly Father.
>
> You reach up and grab that hand. You're out of the box—into a beautiful field. There are trees nearby. There's a brook nearby. The sky is blue and the grass is very, very green and very, very comfortable. You can be by yourself or you can have others join you. But you're very happy and you're very, very peaceful. And you feel really good about yourself.
>
> As you start to turn around, you notice that your box has become bigger. You begin to recognize that you can alter that box. You can put windows in it and you can put a door in it. You can come and go at will. You can rest in it. You can feel comfortable in it, recognizing that, yes, it's still there, but now you have some influence over what you can do with that box.
>
> Okay, let's go inside the box and you can find out. You can imagine that you have two warm heat lamps over each hand and you begin to feel your hands get warmer and warmer. You almost think that you're at the beach and the sun is beating down on your hands and it's getting almost too warm. In fact, they're feeling sweaty, it's so warm, so warm. But you feel very peaceful and very comfortable and very relaxed.

So this has been a session of traveling that can make you feel more relaxed and more at peace. And now before you open up your eyes, you slowly count 1, 2, 3, 4, 5, and you are feeling happy and peaceful and very, very calm. And you open your eyes.

Diana then has the class stretch and "wake up" slowly, because, as she explains to them, their external blood vessels are probably dilated and their internal ones constricted. Getting up too rapidly might make them a little light-headed. She uses this exercise with people of all ages, even very young children.

Now we're going to introduce you to another guide, to someone who can individually help you, to a very wise advisor. It's a person who knows much more about you than we ever could. Here's how you go about meeting this advisor.

Think about a calm and beautiful place, a place where you have been contented and at ease. It could be in the mountains or beside the sea or a lake or a stream or in the desert or the woods, anywhere that you feel in harmony with yourself and the world.

Close your eyes and go there. Visualize yourself walking into this calming place. Hear the sounds, smell the aromas, touch the foliage or the sand or the grass, feel the warmth or the coolness. Experience it with body and mind. Sit down and rest for a while, enveloped by the peace.

Gradually become aware that you are not alone. There is someone sitting nearby. It is a person who is wise and kind, all-knowing, all-understanding, all-forgiving. Perhaps it's someone out of your past—your grandmother or grandfather, an aunt or uncle, a teacher or counselor. Or perhaps it's someone you've never met—and yet you know each other. You know you can rely on this person to help you.

You smile at your advisor. Your advisor smiles back. You talk for a while. You ask if you can have help in finding some answers. Your advisor says, "Of course."

You ask a question. Perhaps it's not the most important question of your life at this early stage of your relationship, but still it's an important question. Wait for the answer. Give your advisor time to think and respond. Your advisor *will* respond.

Continue to sit calmly and think about what you have been told, with all of its possible meanings.

When you feel you have truly understood the message, thank your advisor and embrace him or her warmly before you depart. Say that you look forward to returning and talking again soon.

As you leave your peaceful place, you feel joyful, fulfilled, healthy, loving, and that most nebulous and sought-after of conditions, happy.

Visit your peaceful place and your advisor until all your life questions are answered. You will discover what changes you need to make and you will have the courage and strength to make them.

Perhaps you have already figured out who this advisor really is: your own inner wisdom. After all, only you have the knowledge and insight to answer the important questions you're going to be asking about yourself and your life. With guided imagery you can open a wonderful new communication between your conscious and unconscious minds and solve many problems, including your diabetes problems, through your own creativity.

SOME TIME FOR YOURSELF

With all of these unstressing techniques the most important, and the hardest, part is taking the time to do them. Sometimes it doesn't matter so much which method you choose as that you get out from under your routines and pressures and demands while you're practicing whatever method you prefer.

Some quiet moments alone just doing five minutes of deep abdominal breathing (inhale for a count of four, hold for eight, exhale for eight) can help. So can good old-fashioned daydreaming. Let your mind roll on to whatever pleasant spot you like and picture yourself doing whatever pleasant activity you most enjoy. You have to learn how to escape from the demands of others and carve out time for yourself to do these therapies.

You must have heard by now the basic psychological truth that before you can love others you have to love yourself. There are other related truths for you as a diabetic to remember. You have to take in order to be able to give. You have to be selfish in order to be selfless. You have to help yourself in order to be the most help to others.

Help yourself out of your problems and into a good and healthy life.

PART III
A Blithe Spirit

On June 9, 1979, at the American Diabetes Association annual meeting in Los Angeles a couple of very unorthodox wonder drugs for diabetics were introduced in a lecture to a luncheon gathering. These drugs had only been tested anecdotally rather than in controlled studies with laboratory mice, and the two persons who developed and introduced them were not scientists or licensed professionals in the field of diabetes. Before the presentation was over, however, the physicans, nurses, dietitians, educators, and executives of the ADA were all partaking of these wonder drugs themselves and giving every indication of wholeheartedly endorsing them as efficacious in a program of diabetes care.

These two unorthodox drugs (as well as two others discovered since then) are vitually guaranteed to bring about the third part of your diabetes health triumvirate, a blithe spirit. And just what are these wondrous wonder drugs? They are travel, pets, laughter, and hugs.

None of these drugs has harmful interactions, but they do potentiate one another for the better. We recommend that you add all four of these to your diabetes therapy program. No prescription required.

CHAPTER 10
Travel

When June was in the throes of those chronic headaches we described earlier, she noticed a strange phenomenon. Any time she went on a vacation the headaches disappeared instantly. It was truly remarkable. On plane flights hardly had the wheels left the tarmac when poof! a headache that had been clamped to her skull for a week let go and floated away—and stayed away for the extent of the trip. Then upon her return home, it reappeared.

Some of June's acquaintances offered the theory that because she didn't have headaches on vacations, she must not like her work. She was obviously drumming up headaches as an excuse to get away from it. This was absolutely untrue and we knew it. She loved her work at the Valley College Library and was never in her life a malingerer.

We developed another theory. It must be the foul and fetid air in Los Angeles that caused the headaches, since as soon as she got into the pressurized cabin of an airplane where the air was different, her headaches left. We offered this theory to one of the many doctors she was seeing at the time to try to cure the headaches. This doctor, an expert in sinus problems, said that the air could possibly be the cause. Many of his patients, he said, were affected adversely by the smog. In desperation June moved to the desert where the air was clean, or at least cleaner. That worked for a few months, but then the headaches came back. She then moved to Laguna Beach, California, to see if sea air made a difference. Same story as above.

At this time, a headache specialist finally discovered the True Cause of June's headaches: TMJ (temporomandibular joint) syndrome. This is a malfunction of the jaw hinge joint. When that joint is off-kilter it sets off pain that can wind up in any part of the body—leg, back, head. Why would the TMJ pain be any different on a vacation than at home? When she was at home and at work—with all the built-in stresses and problems of those two locations—she unconsciously clenched her teeth (day and night) and that set off the pain. On a vacation, away from those stresses, she didn't clench and didn't get the headaches.

They always say that you can't leave your troubles behind when you go on a trip. They are wrong! We find you *can* leave them behind, and the farther you're away from them the better. You realize you can't do anything about your problems from this distance, so you finally put them out of your mind and decide just to relax and enjoy yourself. The stress-reduction techniques we described before are like mental mini-vacations. The real thing works even better.

Now while you probably don't have TMJ syndrome, you *do* have diabetes; and literally getting away from your daily stresses can make your diabetes easier to control. Sometimes almost too easy. June has found that on a vacation when she's relaxed, her blood sugars start dropping hazardously and she either has to cut back on her insulin or eat more. This happens to her almost as quickly as getting rid of the headaches in the past.

IN TRAINING FOR TRAVEL

William F. Buckley once said that good training for the sport of yacht racing would be to stand in an ice-cold shower tearing up dollar bills. What with rising costs and—in the case of foreign travel—the falling dollar, the second part of that training session might work for travel as well.

But seriously, folks, for a successful trip some training is essential. The best training, of course, is a lifetime of travel experience. It's always sad to see people who save up their travel for when they retire, planning to take a "Really Big" trip then. More often than not, they cut out on the trip early because they're not enjoying themselves since they're not in training, not used to the inevitable vicissitudes of travel.

So the first piece of advice is TRAVEL NOW. Don't wait. And certainly don't use your diabetes as an excuse to delay. Your diabetes is going to be a lifelong companion, so teach it early on to be a good travel companion.

Dry Run

If you haven't done much travel—especially after the advent of diabetes—before launching on a major excursion you should take a small weekend trip to someplace nearby. Pack all your diabetes supplies and any other health supplies you may use. (*Tip:* Get one of those plastic cosmetic bags with zippered compartments and a hook for hanging. These can be rolled up and tied for easy packing and unrolled and hung up on a shower curtain rail or towel rack. Mark all the compartments to indicate what's in each. When we travel together, we have one with compartments marked "June," "Barbara," "Mutual," and [the biggest one] "Diabetes.")

On your dry run, experiment with the comfort and wrinkleability of your wardrobe. See if you have everything you need to wear. And just as important, see what items you can get along without. Build up your confidence about eating out three meals a day. Then, when the real trip comes, you know exactly how to pack and unpack and most of all to enjoy yourself.

Companion

Diabetes is a companion you can't travel without. All others are optional. As Hemingway said in *A Moveable Feast*, "Never travel with someone you don't love." We even know some devoted husbands and wives who can't travel together because each has a diametrically opposite idea of what a vacation should be. Test out your travel companion on that dry run just as carefully—or even more so—than your wardrobe.

Do you have the same rhythms of life? Are you both morning or evening people? Do you both like a tidy room or a messy one? And—this is vital—do you have a similar sense of humor, particularly an appreciation for the ridiculous?

You must also give your travel companion a crash course in diabetes so that he or she will be able to handle emergencies. See if the person can be relaxed about the situation. If someone looks terrified at the very thought of a diabetic emergency, shop for another companion. You also might shop for things that abort emergencies. For example, one friend of ours, Laura, almost lost her best travel companion when she passed out during a midnight hypoglycemia attack. The friend was so frightened that she refused to travel with Laura because it might happen again. Laura solved the problem by getting a Sleep Sentry to beep her awake before her blood sugar started plummeting. Insulin-takers shold always stock plenty of blood-sugar-raising snacks as well as glucose tablets like Dextrosols and one of the gels like InstaGlucose or Glutose.

Footwork

An army may travel on its stomach, but tourists travel for the most part on their feet. That's why for an agreeable trip you need comfortable feet and legs in good muscle tone. Before your trip, get two pairs of comfortable walking (or running) shoes. Break them in with a gradually increasing walking program.

Try to get up to three or four miles at once before you leave. Also be sure you do some of your walking in hilly areas and practice climbing lots of stairs. The socks we recommend are the Double Lay-R socks endorsed by Dr. Peter Lodewick in *A Diabetic Doctor Looks at Diabetes.* We stock these at the Sugar-Free Centers. They are not only tremendously comfortable but also prevent blisters because the layers rub against one another when you walk instead of one layer rubbing against your foot.

Airport

Whether your travel is foreign or domestic, you'll probably spend a lot of time in airports what with all the delayed and canceled flights. If you *really* want to train for travel, go out and spend twelve hours in a local airport. Bring along food enough for a couple of meals—or try to piece nutritious meals together from the airport eateries. (Real challenge, that one!) Practice sleeping on a bench or propped up in the corner of one. Learn to amuse yourself with crossword puzzles or a book or by chatting with other delayed travelers. Load your syringes and shoot in darkened restrooms. Develop your aplomb at taking blood sugars in public. Learn how to get into what marathon runner Frank Shorter calls his "travel mode" in which you stay relaxed and let nothing bother you. (As we keep emphasizing, stress shoots up your blood sugar faster than pecan pie!)

Financial Training

Another stress reducer is understanding your money (in foreign travel), knowing how to tip, and being certain that you've brought enough money for your needs. Your bank or Deak & Company (offices in most major cities) can arrange for you to get foreign bills and coins for the countries you're visiting. You can practice making change at home. Both at home and abroad you should learn to tip appropriately. (Tipping even differs slightly in U.S. cities; for example, 20 percent is what cab drivers in New York City expect for a tip, and nobody wants to upset a New York City cab driver!)

In figuring how much money to take, remember that travel is like doing house renovations. You work out an estimate with your contractor (travel agent). Then you figure it's going to be half again or twice as much. So start tearing up those dollar bills and you'll be in perfect travel training.

A GRAB BAG OF UNORTHODOX TRAVEL RULES

You've probably read the basic travel rules for diabetics (take double supplies and a prescription for everything, keep supplies with you at all times, take two pairs of comfortable shoes, take diabetes I.D. in English and languages of countries visited, and so on) so often that you'll feel you need to take dramamine if you hear them one more time. That's why we're digging deep into our collective travel reticule to try to come up with some slightly different but equally important rules for a happy, healthy, and successful trip.

We can't take credit for the first two rules. They were conceived by a nondiabetic foreign correspondent, which just goes to show that rules for a diabetic are often not that different from Everyperson.

Always go to the bathroom whenever you can. This means go when there's an opportunity—whether you really need to or not. In travel you never know when the opportunity will present itself again. In foreign travel this is particularly important. It's not that easy to find restrooms overseas. *The New York Times* 'Travel' section recently featured a whole article on how to find a restroom in Rome, thus acknowledging that it's a real challenge. Service stations don't always have them and when they do, it's as it was with a friend of ours who stopped at an isolated French service station. He asked where the restroom was. The attendant fixed him with a gimlet eye and asked if he wanted to buy gas. When he said no, he didn't need any gas, the attendant firmly stated, "Pas d'essence; pas de toilette [No gas; no restroom]." Even on home ground, though, this rule should be observed as a safety measure, especially in automobile travel. A psychologist friend told us her doctor brother maintains that in automobile accidents more damage is done by full bladders exploding on impact than by almost anything else. She won't let guests out the door to go home without first visiting the facilities.

Of course, for diabetics, back in the olden days of urine testing, there was a double reason for following the war correspondent's rule. But now since the golden age of blood glucose monitoring is here, you might add to this rule: *Always test your blood sugar whenever you can.* When traveling, you may be going into different time zones and may be either more relaxed or more stressed. You may be more tired than usual. Your body has a lot of unfamiliar sensations and you may not pick up on your usual signals. June usually tests about twice as often when traveling since she wants to be able to catch a falling blood sugar before it gets too low or nip a rising one in the bud. Only by keeping your blood sugar in excellent control can you feel your best on a trip, and it's a shame to waste a trip by not feeling top notch every minute.

If you're traveling by automobile and you're the driver, you should always test before getting behind the wheel, and every time you stop for a restroom break. It's just basic good sense for self-preservation and the preservation of others.

Never take more luggage than you can carry at a dead run for 150 yards. Naturally a war correspondent might have more reason to run than the average traveler, and for most of us carrying a well-loaded travel purse or in-flight bag at a dead run for 150 yards might be more of a challenge than we'd care to take up. But the point is well taken. Don't take more luggage than you can carry yourself because yourself may be the only person around to do it (and you'd *never* want to leave part of your luggage unattended while you carry the other part). In fact, you really shouldn't let your luggage out of your sight, especially that part of it with your diabetes supplies. Just this year two separate sets of friends traveling in Europe had their rental car broken into at high noon parked on a busy street. One was in Aix-en-Provence, the other in Genoa. They just left their cars for a little over an hour while they ate lunch. When they returned they were picked clean, not even a road map left. The police could do nothing but commiserate and shrug—"it happens all the time." These people had to go out and find new clothes, toilet articles, and cameras. Suppose diabetes equipment and supplies had been stolen. Where in Genoa or Aix would you find another meter and strips and your kind of insulin or oral hypoglycemics? And from all the cautionary Karl Malden American Express commercials, you aren't much safer from the brigands in the good old US of A, so always carry your bags with you. But we'll modify the rule to the extent that you don't *have to* carry them at a dead run.

Assume any plane you take will be late. The old adage, "If you've time to spare, go by air" has never been more true. Since deregulation in this country, flights have become more and more unreliable in their take-off time. Flights are so irregular now that your travel agent can call up on his or her computer the arrival-time statistics for each flight, thanks to a new government regulation. It is even said that most airlines have two schedules: the one they advertise and the actual one used by the airline personnel, which is almost invariably later.

This is significant for a diabetic in many ways. Meal times can be thrown off and your system can be calling for food when the airline is announcing another delay in take-off time. There may be no food available in the airport, or the airport is so crowded with other delayed flight people that you can't get to it. If you must travel at a time when you will be needing a meal, to be on the safe side you should bring plenty of food with you. Then your only problem will be how to avoid the doglike hungry stares of your fellow travelers who are not so well prepared.

Delayed flights can cause an extreme stress response very detrimental to your blood sugar: as the adrenalin you're pumping signals your liver for fight or flight, it sends out the sugar to give you the energy to fight or flee. Since under the circumstances you can do neither, you just sit there with mounting blood sugar. The stress is lessened if you've taken our advice and already assumed the flight is going to be late. You haven't tried to make close connections with another flight because you know in advance you couldn't possibly arrive in time for one. You've probably even decided in advance to stay overnight and catch the continuing flight the next morning. Then if some miracle occurs and the flight *is* on time, you can consider it a thrilling surprise and a bonus to your trip.

Upgrade whenever and however you can. Most articles on travel try to tell you how to pinch pennies and find rock-bottom travel bargains. Often following this advice, you can wind up in uncomfortable situations (*translation:* flea bags and greasy spoons) that wear you out, spoil your trip, and run down your health. Don't get us wrong—we believe firmly in bargains, but what we like are *upgrade bargains.* These are arrangements whereby you can have something really nice, maybe even wonderful, for the price of something basic. There are more of these appearing every day as the competition for the tourist dollar increases. If you're a regular flyer, you undoubtedly already know about joining up with the various airlines for their frequent flyer bonuses. Although it takes an awful lot of air miles to get a free ticket, upgrades to business or first class don't take nearly as many. There are also other ways to get airline upgrades. For example, Williams-Sonoma, a gourmet kitchenware company, once had an intriguing offer in its mail-order catalog: order any product from them and for $25 more they would sell you a TWA upgrade coupon. You could use this to upgrade any rock-bottom tourist ticket on the airline to business class or, if the plane didn't have a business class, first class. You can bet we placed our orders for that one. We've heard people question the value of business or first class for a diabetic who can't eat all that food and certainly can't drink all that alcohol. True. But you can stretch out and sleep in all that seat and arrive ten times more refreshed and ready for action than if you had been sardinized in the tourist section of a full plane. And, as for the food, true you can't eat it all, but you can eat what you want when you want it. When the flight attendants have just a few people in first and business class to take care of, they can cater to their individual needs. So although we'll seldom—if ever—pay the inflated prices for these higher classes, we'll comb newspapers and magazines (and catalogs!) to find all the special upgrading deals we can. We're planning to issue a "See Our World" section in the *Health-O-Gram* from time to time to announce such upgrade bargains as well as some of our favorite travel destinations.

But it isn't just on airlines that you can get luxury for the price of basic. In major cities the best hotels offer special weekend packages that work out to be much less than their weekday rates when the hotel is full of business people. On these weekend specials they often throw in a few other goodies—like a meal in their restaurant and fruit in the room. Ask your travel agent about these specials and look through the travel section of major city newspapers. By the way, these weekend specials aren't just in this country. On a recent trip we found they were available in both Paris and London, making those two horrendously expensive cities only terribly expensive.

Your Diabetic Passport

We mentioned that diabetes is a companion that you can't travel without. It can be a boon companion.

The first thing to remember is to be totally accepting of your diabetes. Never hide it or act embarrassed about it. Since we're always up-front about June's diabetes, it has given us some pleasant adventures and allowed us to get acquainted with some wonderful people.

In *The Peripatetic Diabetic,* we reported how—when we were in Sri Lanka and visited a Buddhist temple in Mount Lavinia—a diabetic priest became so excited when he learned that June was diabetic that he went racing back to his quarters to get his oral hypoglycemic to show her. He then gave us a wonderful personal tour of the temple.

One night in San Francisco we were dining in Trader Vic's. The room was dark, as Trader Vic's often tends to be. June didn't feel like trying to find the restroom to take her shot, so she just asked Barbara to discreetly give it to her in her arm. Later when the maître d' came by to take the order, he said he had noticed what we were doing. He explained that he too was a diabetic and then spent time carefully going over the menu with us, explaining which dishes to avoid because they contained honey or sugar.

One of our favorite diabetic adventures took place in New York. Years ago when Barbara read the Dan Jenkins book, *Semi-Tough,* she became intrigued by the repeated mention of bacon cheeseburgers at P. J. Clarke's (on Third Avenue at 55th Street). Her later study of New York City guidebooks revealed that P. J. Clarke's is supposed to be a hang-out of the New York publishing and advertising set. Since that's the kind of people she likes to share atmosphere with, Barbara always insists on going there at least once every trip to New York, preferably the first night. (Yes, yes, we know that bacon cheeseburgers are hardly the kind of low fat/high fiber fare we've been raving about, but once a year doesn't hurt. *Remember the motto:* Moderation in all things—including moderation!)

On our most recent trip to New York we arrived at the hotel around dinner time. June wanted to take her insulin in the hotel before going to the restaurant—at P. J. Clarke's the restroom facilities are not exactly palatial and brilliantly lit. Since it was Friday, we knew there might be trouble getting a table. Barbara called for a reservation and became engaged in the following conversation with the maître d':

"Would you have a table for two in about fifteen minutes?"

"I think we could fit you in about then."

"Are you sure? You see, I have to know because I'm a diabetic and I'm taking my insulin right now and I have to be certain I can eat without too much delay." (Barbara often claims to be the diabetic. It takes any burden and embarrassment and *boredom* of having to say it off June, and since she isn't diabetic, she feels free about blurting it out. Other friends and family members of diabetics should try it.)

"Isn't that a coincidence?" said the voice on the line. "I just took my insulin, too. And, yes, you can be *sure* you'll get a table right away."

We weren't there two minutes before the genial maître d', whose name we later learned was James (for privacy we'll leave off the last name), escorted us to a table and made certain that we got attentive, friendly, and *fast* service. On our return to California we sent him a *Health-O-Gram* to encourage him to take good care of his diabetes. Now, every time we go to New York, we feel we have a home and a friend at P. J. Clarke's—and all because of diabetes.

We've also met a lot of interesting, receptive people on planes. If June is going to take her injection at her seat—or Barbara is going to give it to her—we always explain to our seat mate what we're going to do and invite him or her to look away if it might be disturbing. This has been a great ice-breaker. Almost every person we've encountered has a diabetic family member or friend and is interested in discussing the subject. One seat mate turned out to be a nurse, who criticized Barbara's injection technique because she didn't aspirate (pull back on the syringe to see if there was blood). This led to a lively exchange about whether or not aspiration is necessary. (We—and most diabetes nurse educators—contend that it isn't.)

These are just a few examples of the doors that the key of diabetes can open for you in travel. Don't keep it hidden in your purse or pocket, and you too can unlock many new and pleasant experiences.

Cautionary Note: Some people are allergic to even the most wonderful of wonder drugs. There are those who have an awful reaction to penicillin. There are those who get stomach distress from aspirin. And, sad for us to have to say, there are those few people who are allergic to travel. They just flat out don't like it, maybe even hate it. Although (as you may have gathered) we're not the slightest bit allergic to this wonder drug ourselves, we can understand their adverse reaction. Travel can be hard work. Travel can be frustrating. Travel can be exhausting. At times travel can wear down your health and upset your diabetes. For those of us for whom travel is as much of a life necessity as work, love, and oxygen, there's no problem at all with the trade-off. We hop to it without batting an eye. But if you're only traveling because someone else wants you to or because it's in style and everybody's doing it, you should stay at home and cultivate your garden or build a beautiful piece of furniture or do whatever it is you most like to do. Otherwise you're likely to wake up some night at 3:00 A.M. in a far-off somewhere, lying on a lumpy mattress, listening to someone trying to start a motorcycle outside your window, your stomach burning with indigestion from the strange food, your feet aching from a day of treading the cobblestones, starting to feel the raspy beginnings of a sore throat, while you wonder if your blood sugar is low—or high—but you feel too tired to get up and test it, asking yourself "How did I get into this?" We'd hate to have you say June and Barbara did it with their travel wonder-drug pushing. No, if you are definitely allergic to travel, then leave it on the shelf for others. After all, we still have three other wonder drugs for you.

CHAPTER 11
Pets

Before Amy Miller, one of our diabetic employees, left the SugarFree Center to have her perfect baby, Andrew, she used to bring in her perfect beagle, Lester, every Wednesday afternoon. He spent his time in the patio off the reception area where he was clearly visible to everyone who came in. Some of these people who came in were not in the greatest frame of mind because they had just been diagnosed diabetic and were scared and worried. On top of that, they may have been told to go out and learn how to stick their fingertips and take blood sugars and spend money they didn't want to spend on a machine they didn't want to buy to control a disease they didn't want to have. No, they weren't feeling too great. But if their eye chanced to fall on Lester, they usually smiled in spite of themselves. Often, after ascertaining that he was friendly, they would go out and talk to him and scratch him behind a floppy ear. You could tell they felt a lot better. We called Lester our pet therapist, deciding that in some cases he did patients more good than the most learned of diabetologists.

Athough we accidentally discovered Lester's therapeutic benefits, our later reading and research revealed that pets truly do wonders for people's physical and mental well-being.

Dr. Elliot Joslin in the original *Joslin's Manual* gave a tribute to how much dogs have done for diabetics. He pointed out that not only did dogs help in the discovery of insulin but a dog is always ready to go for a walk with you. As you know from the exercise section, this is great for your diabetes control. Joslin also said that, best of all, a dog will never lap up some delicious dish that isn't on your diet and then proceed to tell you how fabulous it was—the way some people do.

A dog can even save your life. At least one saved Candy Sangster's life. Candy is a longtime friend of ours at the SugarFree Center. One day she came in to tell us that her dog Jet had been nominated for the Ken-L Ration Dog Hero of the Year Award. She gave us a copy of the nomination write-up.

Dog's name:	Gridiron's Air Coryell (after Don Coryell, NFL Coach)
Nickname:	Jet
Breed:	Doberman Pinscher
Gender:	Female
Age:	6 years
Weight:	75–80 pounds
Dog's favorite activities:	Riding in the van with her head hanging out the window; spending time with her owners
Date of heroic deed:	October 31, 1986
Owners:	George and Candy Sangster

Around dinner time on Halloween, Hazel Lavin heard a dog barking. It was Jet, the Doberman Pinscher, belonging to her next-door neighbors, George and Candy Sangster. Hazel looked out the window, saw nothing irregular, and returned to what she was doing. When the barking didn't stop, Hazel looked out the window again and saw Jet was in her front yard. She became worried. Jet wasn't the kind of dog who barked a lot. Stranger still, the Sangsters had trained Jet never to leave their yard without them. Hazel wondered how the dog had opened the gate without help. She then noticed that the Sangsters' front door was open and that the lights were on. She called Candy Sangster on the phone, letting it ring repeatedly. When no one answered, thinking something must be wrong, she called the emergency number, 911.

As soon as the paramedics arrived, Jet ran frantically between the driveway and the Sangsters' front door. She looked over her shoulder and waited for them. Hazel and the paramedics agreed that Jet seemed to be motioning them inside. The paramedics were a little apprehensive—Jet was, after all, a Doberman. But she wouldn't give up. Finally, with her eloquent dog body language, she convinced them to follow her into the house.

They found Candy Sangster on the living room floor, unconscious. A diabetic, Candy had passed out earlier in the evening with severe hypoglycemia. As the paramedics worked feverishly to bring Candy around, Jet stood protectively by her side.

If not for Jet, the paramedics said, Candy would not have lived through the weekend because her husband was out of town and not due back until Sunday, so no one would have been there to find her and call for help. Jet was the paws-down winner of the Ken-L Ration award!

But it isn't just dogs that work as wonder drugs. It's *all* pets. Cuddling a pet or even just watching one calms you down and lowers your blood pressure. A study at the University of Pennsylvania found that the survival rate for coronary patients was better for those with pets. Three deaths occurred among the fifty-three patients who were pet owners and eleven deaths among the thirty-nine who didn't own pets.

A pet can also give an older person who lives alone a new leash on life. People in rest or convalescent homes who were in the depths of despair and wouldn't talk or interact with others often opened up in the presence of an animal. The Hillhaven Convalescent Hospital in Orange County, California, found that Mutty, who is part golden retriever, drew out an elderly man with Alzheimer's disease as no person could.

Janet Ruckert, a psychologist practicing in West Los Angeles, accidentally discovered the value of pet therapy when she had her cat, Clancy, in the office with her because she hadn't had the time before work to drop him off at the vet's for a defleaing. When a little girl with whom Dr. Ruckert had been making no headway started petting Clancy, she began to reveal her real feelings about her father, who had recently divorced her mother and moved away to start a new family.

Another time, Dr. Ruckert's rottweiler puppy, Lorelei, was in the office with her because she felt she was too young to be left at home alone. Lorelei trotted over and nudged a high-powered executive woman patient with whom Dr. Ruckert had been making little progress. When, at Lorelei's insistence, the patient started petting her, she was able to let down her barriers and express the softer side of her nature, her vulnerabilities, and her needs.

After these accidental encounters, Dr. Ruckert decided there was something to this and incorporated pets into certain of her therapy sessions. "Animals are natural therapists," she explains. "During a session not only does their presence allow a patient to express deep emotions and psychological needs more easily, but at home they are warm and sympathetic listeners." Dr. Ruckert is such a believer in the efficacy of pets that she's written a book entitled *The Four-Footed Therapist.* In it she describes what she calls "petcology"—the value of using the relationship of pets and people to improve everyday life.

A pet can be especially important to a diabetic child or teenager who may fear rejection because of being "different." There's nothing like unqualified face-licking love to make you feel good about yourself. If you have no space for a cat or dog, have a cruel landlord who forbids them, or are allergic to animal fur or dander, a bird or a turtle or a tank of fish can provide calming comfort and—very important—something to love and care for and relate to. (A paper delivered in 1981 at the International Conference on the Human-Companion Bond in Philadelphia even describes the value of watching tropical fish to reduce blood pressure.)

The living thing you love and care for doesn't even have to be an animal or bird or turtle or fish to help you with your physical and mental health. A poignant documentary film a few years back told of a lonely woman's love for a green bean plant she had growing in her window. When the plant died at the end of the film, as June put it in her mixed cliché way, "There wasn't a dry tear in the house."

So be it animal or vegetable (not mineral—pet rocks just won't do it), get a pet. Your diabetes and your life will be better with one or more of these wonder drugs.

P.S. We follow our own prescription as Mishka, Little Ngo, Greystoke, and Greystone will attest.

CHAPTER 12
Laughter

We once received what could loosely be described as a fan letter from a reader of our book *The Peripatetic Diabetic.* The letter ended with, "I'm sorry, but I just don't find diabetes as much fun as you two seem to." We thought about that one for a while and then Barbara was assigned to write the response. (Since she doesn't have diabetes, she finds it a mite more fun than June does.)

Barbara wrote our correspondent that we feel that diabetics are well aware of the dismals of the disease. There's no need to have those dismals driven home to them in books and lectures. They have to live with them every day of their lives.

We feel it's our job to help diabetics look on the bright side and find humor and fun and laughter wherever they can, even in the diabetic state and its therapies. A humorist once said, "Just because I laugh at life doesn't mean I don't take it seriously." Just because we laugh at diabetes from time to time doesn't mean we don't take it seriously, and it certainly doesn't mean we don't want *you* to take it seriously. We just want you to keep your sense of humor alive because it's virtually impossible to have a humorous attitude toward something and at the same time to feel angry and resentful toward it.

Psychologist Dr. David Bresler of the UCLA Pain Control Unit says that he always wishes he could check a patient's serum fun level because those patients with a high serum fun level have a much better prognosis for recovery. "We want to make sure our patients have enough fun to break their negative life attitudes," he says.

One of the reasons laughter is such an effective diabetes therapy is that it's a great stress reducer. As Dr. Raymond Moody pointed out in his book *Laugh after Laugh: The Healing Power of Humor*, when you laugh you briefly lose muscle tone. All the tense muscles of the body are relaxed and you have what the British philosopher Herbert Spencer called "a discharge of nervous excitement." Dr. Moody reported that one physician friend found he could cure tension headaches simply by getting patients to laugh at him. Another physician found that all his very healthy elderly patients had one thing in common—a good sense of humor. All in all, Dr. Moody said, he had "encountered a surprising number of instances in which, to all appearances, patients have laughed themselves back to health, or at least have used their sense of humor as a very positive adaptive response to their illness."

Laughter, according to Norman Cousins, the former editor of the *Saturday Review*, is a kind of "internal jogging" that can be even more health restoring than the external kind. Cousins is, in fact, living proof of the healing power of laughter.

He was lying in a hospital bed in agony, suffering from a collagen disease (a disease of the body's connective tissues) that a whole battery of experts couldn't cure. One day Cousins accidentally saw a letter his doctor had written to a mutual friend. In it appeared the sentence, "I'm afraid we're going to lose Norman." That did it. He decided it was time for him to get involved in his own case.

Since he knew that negative emotional states can make a person susceptible to illness, he reasoned that positive emotion might help bring about recovery. And what, he thought, is more positive than a good, straightforward, uncomplicated belly laugh? Cousins arranged to have video tapes of old *Candid*

Camera TV shows played, and lo, after an hour of laughter he found his pain had diminished to such an extent that he could get a good night's sleep. When doctors performed tests on him after one of these laugh sessions, they found that the inflammation in his tissues had lessened.

Another aspect of Cousins' self-therapy that must have done much toward activating his joy gland and increasing his serum fun level was checking out of the hospital, with his doctor's approval, and into a luxury hotel. Not only was the cost considerably lower at the hotel (which contributes a lot to one's good spirits) but the food was more appetizing and the service just as attentive.

The end of the Cousins story is a happy one. He lived to tell the tale of his illness and unusual therapy in the *New England Journal of Medicine* and is now well and strong and giving guest lectures at the UCLA Medical School.

Now it's true that Cousins was also taking large doses of vitamin C, and his cure may have been brought about by that, or maybe it was just a matter of nature taking its course and he would have recovered no matter what he did. Still, deep down in our funny bones, we feel that laughter had a lot to do with it. We also feel that if you increase your own personal supply of this wonder drug it can't help but do good things for your health and your diabetes.

The big question, then, is where do you get a steady supply?

ELIMINATE THE NEGATIVE PEOPLE

Negative people are worse for diabetics than positive urine tests. As the French existentialist Jean-Paul Sartre said, "Hell is—other people!" But that's only half of it. Heaven can also be other people. You just have to find the right people, the positive people, the ones who fill you with joy and laughter rather than gloom and doom.

We have a term for these negative sorts—prana suckers. *Prana* is the Sanskrit word for life force, and after you've been with these people for a while you feel as if they've sucked the life force right out of you the way a vampire sucks blood. You feel totally drained.

One tendency of prana suckers is to be blemish finders. This means they only have eyes for flaws. If you take blemish finders into a room full of beautiful art objects except for one ugly little dirty jar off in a corner, they will ignore all the beauty and, scowling with disgust, say, "Would you just look at that ugly little dirty jar!" Even if you have a wonderful life full of activity, work, and people you love, there are bound to be some blemish finders who will focus on and tsk over your one flawed aspect—your diabetes—never mentioning all the reasons you have for happiness.

Prana suckers also seem to be full of what psychologists call negative expectations. They always know the worst is likely to happen—in fact, it definitely *will* happen—and they love to sit around with you and flip through their catalog of potential disasters. For diabetics there are plenty of potential (yet avoidable) disasters that a person can dwell on if so inclined. And just as it's important not to dwell on them yourself, it's important not to hang around with people who want to dwell on them for you.

We're sorry to have to say it, but even doctors can be prana suckers. June's original doctor was a good example of this. He followed up the diagnosis in this delightful way: "Everything about your life is going to have to change. No smoking. No drinking. You have to watch everything—and I mean everything—you eat from now on. Take this diet sheet. If you don't follow this plan to the letter, you can go blind; you can get gangrene of the feet and have an amputation; and you can get kidney failure and die."

June's headache specialist, on the other hand, was exactly the opposite kind of doctor. His sense of humor was always operative. He was invariably hopeful and positive and, above all, he loved his work. We once saw him at a conference, eyes shining with excitement, describing "the fun and reward of helping a patient." That's the kind of doctor you should seek and find.

Sometimes, unfortunately, the negative people are family members and it's pretty hard to avoid them. But remember, negative people are like stress: it's not so much the people themselves as your reaction to them. You've got to keep their negativism from getting to you. You've got to learn to laugh them off.

One way to keep a happy outlook on life is to give yourself a few rewards along the way. We're not advocating total hedonism as there is no grimmer, harder, more depressing work than incessant pleasure seeking. We do feel, however, that diabetics who keep their noses faithfully to the dual grindstones of work or school and diabetes deserve to take some time out for the little pleasures that can at least bring smiles if not outright laughter.

Shari Silver, a diabetic deputy district attorney in Santa Monica, sometimes plays hooky from the pressures of her job and goes to the drugstore to shop for new nail-polish colors, an activity that always makes her feel good. It makes *us* laugh—and probably her as well—to think that this hard-driving lawyer who strikes terror into opponents' hearts in the courtroom is a secret, hopeless nail-polish junkie.

You hear a lot about taking care of yourself on a sick day. Some diabetics will only let down and relax when they're sick. This is bad psychology as well as bad diabetes therapy. We think you should take an occasional day off when you feel terrific. Do something you especially enjoy and never have time for, even if it's just doing nothing. Whatever you do, you'll be practicing a kind of self-conditioning in which your feeling-well state is reinforced. Then you'll find yourself arranging to have more feeling-well states in the future.

And then there are your hopes and dreams. Often you have to delay your gratification until you get through a work project or finish a college degree or some such, but some people delay their gratification forever. They deny their dreams until it's too late to realize them. June has always had tendencies toward gratification delay, but she's doing better at fighting those tendencies these days. Her biggest dream always was to go on a bike tour of Holland. Finally, in the summer of 1979, she delayed it no longer. And now, with her memory bank full of that trip, she's smiling all the way to the fulfillment of her next dream.

Whatever you do, don't deny yourself your dreams because you're afraid your diabetes might cause some awkward problems. If you believe you can't do something you dream of because you have diabetes, think about Judith Oehler-Giarrantana. She's a nurse and rehabilitation psychologist at Retina Associates in Boston. She's also a blind diabetic. But she didn't let that stop her from becoming the first blind person to complete a rigorous Wilderness Survival course. Try on this quote from her for inspirational size:

> The boat was completely open—no kitchen, bunks, or head (which meant testing urine over the side of the boat.) The first night I didn't do a urine test; it was difficult enough to learn to brush our teeth and take care of toilet needs over the side of the boat. The next day, however, I was comfortable enough to ask others to assist me.

And this:

> The most difficult exercise was the split log. I had to cross two logs, suspended end to end twenty feet in the air, with a four-foot gap in the middle. I crept across, hanging onto a rope with an instructor verbally guiding me. When I got to the gap I crouched down and stretched one foot across it. I had difficulty locating the other log with my foot so I returned to the crouched position to rest. The second time I was successful! After I had finished, one of the instructors told me that was the one exercise they had felt could not be completed by a blind person.

As she summed it up, "Outward Bound reaffirmed for me the necessity of taking meaningful risks in order to reach my full potential." We'll bet that her accomplishment gave her a big smile of personal satisfaction.

THE GREAT PRETENDER

You may think this talk about laughter and smiles and how therapeutic they are is all very well, but what if you don't feel full of fun and optimism with the specter of diabetes continually floating around in your consciousness? Well, then, what you do is just *pretend* you're a happy person.

Kurt Vonnegut had as the moral of his book *Mother Night,* "We are what we pretend to be, so we must be careful about what we pretend to be." Mark that well. Pretend to be a miserable, down-feeling, hopelessly sick person with your joy gland in worse shape than your pancreas and that's what you'll be. Decide to be a healthy, hopeful, vital person and *that's* what you'll be.

To help you get started with your new happy attitude, we'll try to get you laughing with a story from the Prohibition era. It seems there was this drinking gentleman whose regular bootlegger was put out of commission by the Elliot Ness boys. The gentleman quickly found himself another bootlegger, but this bootlegger's product was a little strange-tasting. Since he'd heard stories of people being made sick, or worse, by bootleg whiskey, he decided to be on the safe side and send it to a laboratory for analysis.

The report came back. "Dear Sir," it read. "We're sorry to have to tell you this, but your horse has diabetes."

There, now, didn't that make you feel good?

CHAPTER 13
Hugs

If laughter seems to be an unusual diabetes therapy, this one may strike you as downright outlandish, so we'd better give you a little of the background and scientific rationale of this wonder drug. Its discovery came about when Barbara, who was then a college librarian, read an article in a library publication that told of an experiment at Purdue University. The library workers were instructed to "accidentally" touch the hands of certain students as they were checking out books to them. The touch was to be so brief and light that the student might not even be consciously aware that it was happening.

Then members of the psychology department lurking outside the library would stop the students and interview them. It turned out that the students who had been touched had much warmer, more positive feelings toward the library, toward themselves, and toward life in general than those who hadn't been touched. Why was this so?

Well, as family therapist Helen Colton, author of *The Joy of Touching*, explains, "Our need to be touched, caressed, and cuddled is as basic as our need for food. . . . Without it we get a kind of malnutrition of the spirit."

As you must have noticed, our culture is not big on touching the way Latin and Mediterranean cultures are, so a lot of us are walking around with malnutrition of the spirit. These Purdue University students had for once had their touching needs met, and it was an almost instantaneous change from malnourished to nourished.

Barbara mused on this touching experiment and decided it was just what both the library and the students needed. We could combine great public relations for the library with improved mental health for students—something they especially needed in this era of lowered expectations when there might be no jobs waiting for them on graduation.

She announced to the staff of the check-out desks what she expected them to do. Uptight puritan types that they were, they flatly refused to give students a subtle nourishing touch along with their books. "All right," said Barbara like the Little Red Hen, "then *I* will." But though she had every opportunity to touch when helping students with the periodical indexes, she couldn't bring herself to do it. It somehow seemed sneaky and furtive to be "accidentally" brushing against students' hands. The good idea appeared to die a-borning.

But then, about this time, we were talking to Dr. David Bresler of the UCLA Pain Control Unit in conjunction with our headache book. Dr. Bresler said that chronic pain is sometimes a subconscious cry for love and tender treatment. Because people can't bring themselves to march up to someone and say directly what they want, they announce a pain (a real pain) to elicit the sympathy, the soothing touch they need. This is why one prescription that Dr. Bresler always gives his chronic-pain patients is four hugs a day. He considers these hugs so important that he even advises patients who don't have a huggee handy to approach strangers in the supermarket and hug them.

That suddenly clicked with Barbara. Hugs are even better than touches. They're more up-front, with nothing sneaky or furtive about them.

Back in the library she posted a sign on the suggestion board explaining the value of touching and hugging (lest the students consider her some kind of nut) and offering herself as hug therapist. She invited all students to drop by her desk for hug therapy whenever they had a need.

She pinned on the hug-therapist badge she'd made for herself and waited. And waited and waited. A week. Nothing. Two weeks. Still nothing. It began to look as if the hug-therapy program was also destined to trickle down the drain to oblivion.

Then one morning Barbara looked up to find a young man standing in front of her desk. He cleared his throat, and swallowed. "Are you Barbara Toohey?"

"Yes."

"Well . . . er . . . ah . . . I think I could use a hug."

Barbara almost tripped over the wastebasket getting to him. They clutched each other awkwardly, blushing to the tops of their ears. But do you know what? They both felt wonderful afterward. Maybe it was partly the result of surviving a difficult ordeal, but more likely it was the hug, the human contact, the reaffirmation of identity and self-worth.

This first hug was like the first olive out of the bottle. The rest came easily. Large numbers of students and faculty members started coming into the library for their hugs. The hugging business got so brisk, especially around finals, that June and the other librarians were pressed into service as surrogate hug therapists. Several students placed themselves on a regular daily hug schedule.

Somehow the media got hold of hug therapy. (It was about the time of the Jonestown massacre and they were hungry for good news.) Hug therapy as practiced in the Los Angeles Valley College Library was on radio and TV and in the newspapers. Hugs had made a minor sweep of the Southern California.

As we worked more and more with hug therapy it gradually dawned on us that this wonder drug, which is so curative for chronic-pain patients and salubrious for students, would be ideal for diabetics. In the first place, since hugging fosters a feeling of self-worth, it makes you more accepting of yourself as you are, diabetes and all. By helping you realize that you are a good person—a *huggable* person—it makes you want to take better care of that good person in order to keep that good person on the planet as long as possible. Hugging also diminishes anger—a very common emotion among diabetics—and, here we go again, it reduces stress. You can feel the tensions flow out of your body in the warmth of a hug.

We believe it would be wonderful if doctors would make it a practice to give a hug along with the diagnosis of diabetes. There is no more dismal time in your life than when you hear yourself being given that life sentence to a chronic disease, the full implications of which you can't quite grasp but which nevertheless fills you with fear and uncertainty. A warm, accepting hug would be like a life preserver to hang onto at that moment. It's like the old laying on of hands that doctors used to practice before they starting keeping us all at instruments' distance. The efficacy of laying on of hands might be just the placebo effect, but don't knock placebos. They have no harmful side effects and they often work. Medical science has recently discovered that placebos, like running, activate the body's endorphin system. This "morphine within" can diminish both physical and psychic pain.

As a matter of fact, all members of the diabetes-care team—nurses, dietitians, social workers—should become hug therapists on the side. Actually, hug therapists are needed everywhere in medicine. Once Barbara was visiting a friend in the hospital and forgot to remove her hug-therapist badge from the library. A dismal-looking woman who shared the elevator with her glanced at the badge and, apparently thinking Barbara was part of the hospital staff, asked, "Hug therapist? What kind of thing is that?" When Barbara explained it to her she said, "I think I'll have one." Barbara hugged her and a good measure of the gloom left the woman's face.

Hugs aren't good merely for your mental health, either. As with all the therapies we've mentioned, the mind can change the body in mysterious and wonderful ways. A recent radio report on this phenomenon amazed even us. Researchers at

Ohio State University were doing a study of how diet affects atherosclerosis. As one of their experiments they fed several groups of rabbits an extremely high-fat diet. Students were assigned to take care of these rabbits. One young woman became so fond of those in her charge that she dropped in several times a day just to pick them up and pat and squeeze them.

At the end of the experiment it was discovered that although the rabbits in her group were eating a diet identical to that of all the other rabbits, her rabbits had only half the fatty deposits in their blood vessels.

Thinking that this was just a strange coincidence, the research team tried the experiment again. Same results. Finally, after repeating the experiment five times, they had to conclude that tender loving care did indeed do something to help prevent atherosclerotic build-up.

Hugs are as beneficial to the hugger as to the huggee. Both of us are sometimes a little shy in first encounters and find that if we announce ourselves as hug therapists and offer our services it breaks the ice better than a cocktail. After all, if you've hugged somebody it's pretty hard to be cool and distant with him or her.

There are, we must admit, a couple of small problems that present themselves in hug therapy. Some people get the wrong idea at first—especially men, who, conditioned by our culture to believe that you are never allowed to touch another person except for sex or violence, find it hard to understand a warm, human, nonsexual encounter like a hug. But we find that most of them are easily indoctrinated and often turn out to be the best huggers of all, probably because they've been deprived for so long. The other problem also concerns men. Men can hug women easily, and women can hug men. Women can also hug other women without difficulty. But, as columnist Ellen Goodman said, "There are men who would die for each other but they can't hug each other." Work on it, men. You need it and so do your friends.

When we started closing our talks to diabetes groups with hug-therapy sessions, it soon became clear that hugs and diabetics are perfect partners. We've even begun to think that, along with bike-a-thons, we should raise funds with hug-a-thons in which you pledge a certain amount of money for each stranger the participant hugs. This would spread salubrious hugs across the nation and, besides helping finance a cure for diabetes, might even prevent diabetes complications. All the blushing that invariably goes on with hugging does tremendous things for your circulation. So get this prescription filled right away:

Rx 4 HUGS A DAY

Hug anyone in the room, anyone in the house, anyone in the library or the office or wherever you are and feel the wonder of this wonder drug.

And to send you on your way, here's one for the road.*

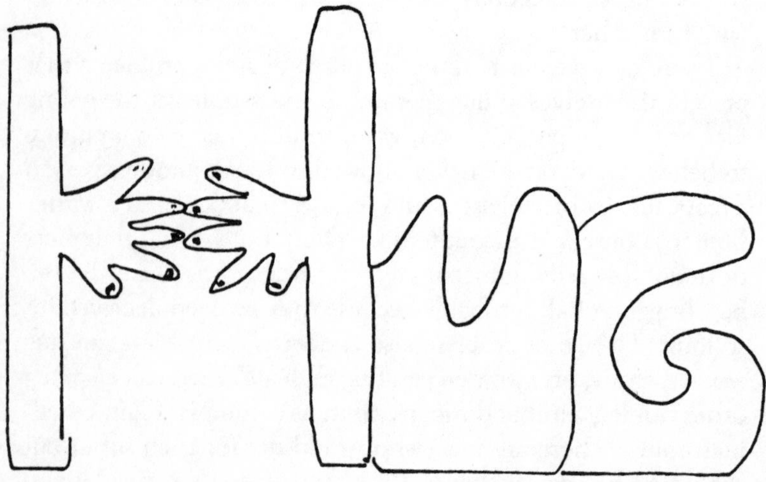

*Courtesy of Janice Kent.

CHAPTER 14
Changes

> "There is no pain in change; there is only pain in resistance to change."
>
> —Judy Collins, *Trust Your Heart*

Now that you've traveled and adopted a pet or two and have laughed and hugged and learned the kinds of changes you can make to bring about total health, it's time to start making those changes. We're not going to tell you that it's easy to change old bad habits to new good ones, to switch from negative addictions to positive ones. Change—even change for the better—produces stress because it takes a lot of effort, and at first it may seem as if you're giving up all that is comfortable and pleasurable in your life.

Maybe it will help if you don't think of it as giving up things, but rather as making trade-offs. Robert Shornick, a diabetic in his fifties writing in *Diabetes Forecast,* expressed the trade-off idea in this way:

> [Diabetes] made me reevaluate how I was spending my time and energy. Such a change demands trade-offs—giving up something in return for something else, not necessarily a negative exchange. Before diabetes, several drinks and a few cigarettes on an airplane after a hectic day was sheer pleasure. Another drink or two in the hotel before bed further relaxed me. Now I have a sugar-free drink on the plane and my food snack at bedtime. Not as

> enjoyable, but adequate. The next day my head is 10 percent clearer than it used to be. A *good trade.*
>
> Before diabetes, my eating habits were erratic, both as to when and what I ate. Now, "when" and "what" have specific meanings for me, and my *energy level has doubled. Therefore, I accomplish more.* A profitable exchange.
>
> Before diabetes, I weighed 158 pounds, looked a bit pudgy, and had difficulty buying suits that fit. Now I weigh 144, am trim and slim, and can find a whole selection from which to choose. *An ego-boosting trade.*
>
> Before diabetes, my exercise pattern was sporadic, heavy on the weekends. Now I exercise daily in a programmed manner, and my body reflects a comfortable tone and hardness.
>
> Before diabetes, much time at home was devoted to necessary business activities to generate income. Now I'm working toward a better balance of work time and family time. My wife and son are the two most important ingredients in my life, so that's where I'm putting a more meaningful share of my life.

There will, of course, always be people who try to sabotage your efforts toward making changes. They will be happy to tell you tales such as the following true story told to June by a friend to whom she had described her new lifestyle with morning jogging and the HCF diet.

This person said he had a friend who had led a freewheeling (translation: self-destructive) life up to his forties, at which time he experienced some sort of midlife crisis and decided all this had to stop. He knew he was wrecking his health with his lifestyle, which was more like a deathstyle. He did an about-face.

He gave up his six-packs and his twenty-packs. He started exercising and worked himself up to a daily five-mile run. He kept regular hours. He ate balanced meals, watching the cholesterol. (As the fellow who told the tale put it, "He gave up everything enjoyable.") He lost weight. Even the tale-teller had to admit grudgingly that his friend looked great. Finally the friend even decided that his old sedentary, high-pressure job, in which he had achieved great monetary success, had to go. He quit and got a physically active outdoor job in construction work. Six months later a wayward steamroller fell on him and killed him.

The tale teller delivered the punch line with a smug, see-all-the-good-it-did-him smile on his face.

But his story did not convince us to ignore the principles of total health, and we hope it won't convince you either. Because—now hear this!—*you cannot count on having a steamroller fall on you.*

Remember the words of comedian Jimmy Durante, who stated on the occasion of his seventy-eighth birthday, "If I'da known I was gonna live dis long, I'da taken better care of myself."

One of our favorite sayings of the greatest diabetologist of them all, Dr. Eliot Joslin, has always been: "Live as if you were going to die tomorrow; learn as if you were going to live forever." But now we realize that this statement is subject to misinterpretation. We assure you that "living as if you were going to die tomorrow" does *not* mean you should follow a heedless eat-drink-and-be-merry philosophy with your health. No, Dr. Joslin meant you should experience life to the fullest. To be able to do that, you have to have the best health you can. In that sense, diabetics need to live and to learn as if they were going to live forever.

Live that way not *just* to keep your diabetes in control. Live that way to have the total health that will enable you to achieve happiness. And what, pray tell, is this nebulous concept of happiness? Philosophers have wrestled with that one for centuries, but no one has yet come up with what is universally accepted as the *definitive* definition. In our opinion the one that comes closest to the mark is Aldous Huxley's. As you set off on the not-always-smooth road to total health, we offer it to you and wish it for you: "Love, peace, joy, and the capacity to help others."

PART IV

An Eclectic Cookbook for Diabetics

The word *eclectic* has many meanings: "selecting or choosing from various sources," "using what are considered the best elements," and "chosen for its fanciful appropriateness." All the meanings apply here.

We've selected and modified these recipes from various sources: favorite cookbooks, favorite national cuisines, favorite restaurants, favorite friends, and favorite successful experiments we've made in the kitchen. Admittedly a few of these recipes may contain a tad more fat than you—or we—normally put in dishes. But these are special treats that you won't be having every day or every week or every month. Even so, don't hesitate to cut back further on fat to stay within your recommended diet. The dishes will still be good.

In the recipes, we use what we consider the best elements—the best ingredients and the best methods of preparation and serving.

We like to think of them all as *fanciful.* The one thing we think food should never be is boring. That's why we've included only dishes that please and tickle our food fancies. We hope they'll do the same for yours.

BASICALLY NOT BASIC

This is by no means a basic cookbook—a complete compendium like the *Joy of Cooking*; or what we consider the diabetic equivalents of that honored tome, *The Art of Cooking for the Diabetic*; or even the four volumes of *The American Diabetes Association/American Dietetic Association Family Cookbooks.*

No, this eclectic collection won't bring you from not knowing how to boil an egg to preparing a state dinner for the prime minister of France. And yet in another sense it *is* basic. We've here tried to explain the recipes in such a way that even a very inexperienced cook could handle them. In some cases where the recipes verge on the time-consuming or complex, we've given a simpler alternative that sacrifices very little in the ultimate enjoyment.

AROUND A DIFFERENT WORLD

In the very first edition of our very first diabetes book, *The Peripatetic Diabetic,* we included an "Around the World Cookbook" including our favorite dishes from different cuisines. We still like international dishes, but the culinary world we explore now is a kinder, gentler-on-your body place with lower fat and sodium and higher fiber. Also, back in those days, when it came to eating out, very expensive French restaurants were about the only place you could find a variety of vegetables prepared in interesting ways. Now our tastes lean toward relatively inexpensive Italian restaurants, and our recipes, with a great emphasis on things Italian, reflect that change of taste. It has been said that when you're in love, the whole world's Italian. It holds equally true that when you're in love with cooking, if the whole world is not Italian, at least a very large part of it is.

PLAY WITH YOUR FOOD

When we encourage you to play with your food, we're not advocating that you draw happy faces in your mashed potatoes or flip spoonfuls of peas at your dining companions. No, we mean that when it comes to cooking, you should be relaxed and happy and make variations on dishes depending on what's in season and what you have in the house.

We ourselves used to be so rigid that when we were making a recipe—especially for the first time—we'd run all over town trying to find exactly the called-for ingredients. Not only did this result in a state of exhaustion and irritation that took away the pleasure of the cooking and eating, but often the dish didn't turn out as well as it would have if we'd played with the recipe using, for example, ingredients that were in season and readily available.

Being flexible with your ingredients is also a thrift measure. What we ordinarily do is take whatever protein (generally the most expensive part of the meal) is on sale and build dinner around that.

Ultimately your greatest fun comes when you become confident and experienced enough in the kitchen to decide you don't want to go out—either to a restaurant or to shop for ingredients—and just make dinner out of what you can find around the house. When you manage to turn out something you've never had before and it's Something Wonderful, your dining pleasure multiplies exponentially.

COME INTO OUR KITCHEN

Now, after this preamble, we invite you to try some of these favorite recipes of ours. We hope you will read them with excitement and anticipation, prepare them—for yourself and others—with love and enthusiasm, and dine upon them with pleasure and joy. For each recipe, we provide you with the nutritional information and diabetes exchanges for one serving of the basic recipe. These were calculated for us by Lambert, DeVito, Bauersfeld and Associates, Registered Dieticians. Optional variations that we suggest or that you make will differ slightly.

However, one of our goals with this little cookbook for diabetics is to free you from feeling you have to use *only* cookbooks for diabetics. We hope that as you work your way through these recipes, you'll start to become familiar enough with ingredients that you will be able to estimate fairly closely what the exchanges are in any and all recipes you may want to try. After all, that's what the exchanges are—fairly close estimations (just as the blood sugar tests you make are only fairly close estimations). To tell the truth, after twenty-five years of following the so-called diabetic diet, we hardly ever use cookbooks specifically designed for diabetics anymore. The one exception we make is when it comes to desserts, which often take quite a bit of delicate balancing of ingredients to deliver the correct texture and sweet taste without excessive calories.

In most cases we've given you the information on how to find special ingredients that we suggest, but if you have trouble locating any of these, write to us at 5623 Matilija Avenue, Van Nuys, CA 91401, and we'll do our best to track them down for you.

BREAKFAST

Most of us prefer something familiar and comforting for the first meal of the day, and that's why we stick to more standard American fare at breakfast. There are few things more familiar and comforting than muffins. We're including two of our favorite recipes here. These are good not just for breakfast, but for a midmorning snack, too.

Breakfast Bran Muffins

Makes 8 muffins

These are our basic breakfast muffins, which June bakes almost every week. Often we even take a batch with us on trips, for breakfast in the hotel room. They are chock full of fiber, and you know how hard it is to get your fiber when traveling—or even at home, for that matter. Miller's bran (not bran cereal) is available in boxes in some supermarkets and in all health-food stores.

1 cup whole wheat flour
3 teaspoons baking powder
½ teaspoon salt (optional)
1 cup bran
2 tablespoons vegetable oil
2 tablespoons Fruit Sweet or molasses
1 egg
1 cup nonfat milk
Raisins (optional)

Heat the oven to 425 degrees. Sift together flour, baking powder, and salt (optional). Add bran and stir thoroughly. In a separate, smaller bowl mix together vegetable oil, Fruit Sweet (available from Wax Orchards; phone 1-800-972-2323) or molasses, the egg, and milk. Add this to the dry ingredients and mix only enough to moisten. Fill Pam-sprayed muffin tins, or tins lined with paper baking cups (we spray these), two-thirds full. Bake for 15 minutes, or until done. As a variation you can add the raisins, either to the whole batch or to half of it.

8 servings Exchanges per serving: 1 starch; 1 fat Calories: 142
Protein: 6 gm Carbohydrate: 23 gm Fat: 5 gm
Fiber: 4 gm Cholesterol: 27 mg Sodium: 268 mg

L.A. Fitness Muffins

Makes about 16 muffins

We call these L.A. Fitness muffins because we keep them in the freezer and have one before going to a workout at our gym (L.A. Fitness Center). But they're really good any *time, and since they have some fruit built in, you can enjoy them* au naturel. *You have your choice of fruit, but do your taste buds a favor and use fresh, not canned, fruit.*

- 1 cup blueberries (or halved cherries, diced peaches, or raspberries)
- 1¾ cups all purpose flour, sifted
- ½ teaspoon salt
- 2 teaspoons double-acting baking powder
- 3 tablespoons granular fructose
- 1 egg
- 1 egg white
- 2 tablespoons avocado or other vegetable oil
- ¾ cup nonfat milk
- 1 teaspoon grated orange or lemon rind

Prepare the fruit first and lightly flour it. Preheat the oven to 425 degrees. Sift together the flour, salt, and baking powder. Add granular fructose and mix thoroughly. In a separate bowl beat the egg and egg white; add avocado oil, milk, and 1 teaspoon grated orange or lemon rind. Add the wets to the dries and blend partially before dropping in the fruit. The entire stirring process should not take more than 20 seconds (there may be some lumps). Fill Pam-sprayed tins two-thirds full; bake 20 to 25 minutes.

16 servings Exchanges per serving: 1 starch Calories: 80
Protein: 2.5 gm Carbohydrate: 12 gm Fat: 2 gm Fiber: 0.6 gm
Cholesterol: 13.5 mg Sodium: 122 mg

You can make wonderful muffins the super-easy way using a prepared blue corn muffin mix available from Natural Choices, Inc. (505-242-3494). They also make a dandy blue corn pancake and waffle mix.

Usually for breakfast, though, we just have cereal of some kind—in warm weather usually a cold cereal such as Fiber I or Breakfast O's (Barbara's Bakery). In cold weather it's oatmeal or oat-bran cereal. We have two favorite oatmeals: McCann's

Irish Oatmeal (the non-quick-cooking variety), which we first discovered when we had breakfast at Rumpelmayers before taking our morning walks in Central Park. (We like to live dangerously!) When time is short you can make a delicious quick-cooking oatmeal that's available from Christine and Rob's (41103 Stayton Scio Road SE, Stayton, OR 97383-9406; phone 503-769-2993). They also have a wonderful old-fashioned baking-powder biscuit mix that makes a lovely Sunday breakfast.

Dr. Ron Brown's Royal Canadian Oat Bran

Serves 1

Oat bran is a little out of style compared with what it was a few years back, but it shouldn't be out of your diet. Just ask Dr. Anderson (see page 57). Not only does oat bran vacuum up cholesterol, but it really sticks to your ribs and every other bone in your body. You feel full for hours, which makes it great for people who are on a weight-losing program.

Dr. Ron Brown, our first employee, is a dietitian as well as a doctor and a magnificent cook. This recipe shows how he took something prosaic and turned it into something really wonderful.

- ⅓ cup oat bran
- ½ cup nonfat milk
- ½ cup water
- Dash salt
- ½ small or ¼ medium green apple
- 1 packet Equal
- 2 dashes cinnamon
- 1 tablespoon roughly chopped peanuts
- 1 tablespoon raisins
- 1 teaspoon sugar-free syrup

Combine oat bran, nonfat milk, water, and salt in a small saucepan. Heat to boiling over medium-high heat. Reduce heat and simmer for 3 minutes. While it simmers, put the following into your cereal bowl: the apple, Equal, cinnamon, peanuts (for half the calories, use Paul's partially defatted, lightly salted, or salt-free peanuts; phone (516) 487-2012), raisins, and sugar-free syrup (Cary's or Diet-Cal). Add cooked oat bran and stir to combine.

1 serving Exchanges per serving: 1 starch; ½ milk; 2 fruit
Calories: 245 Protein: 12 gm Carbohydrate: 47 gm
Fat: 7 gm Fiber: 8 gm Cholesterol: 2.2 mg Sodium: 204 mg

HERBACEOUS LUNCHES

In California we're fortunate that salad greens are easy to come by year round and not hard to grow yourself. People make a lot of fun of Californians and their radicchio and arugula and endive and mache, but in truth these greens do enliven a salad and bring it out of the ordinary. Arugula is the easiest of all to grow yourself, since it's officially classified as a weed, but it's very expensive to buy in the market and even more so in a restaurant. Another easy grower that brightens up the taste of the other greens is mint: chop up a few leaves (not enough to overwhelm) for your mixed green salad and taste the difference. Of course, any other herbs you may have in your garden or pots are welcome: basil, chives, oregano, marjoram, thyme, tarragon. All you need for these salads is a light dressing of oil and vinegar; we like to add a little Dijon mustard to further perk things up.

There are two other slightly more complex salads we particularly enjoy.

A Totally Unauthentic Caesar Salad

Serves 4

Despite arguments to the contrary, Caesar salad was invented in Tijuana, Mexico. We know this for a fact because Barbara was there with her father and had one when she was in junior high. Mexican in origin as it may be, the Caesar salad has been rattling around the United States—especially California—for so long and has gained so much popularity that we've adopted—and adapted—it as our own. Everyone has his or her favorite way of fixing it and claims it to be the most authentic. There is, for example, a raging controversy concerning the inclusion of anchovies. We've heard that Caesar's daughter claims her father would never consider putting anchovies in his. One thing every "authentic" Caesar salad has is a raw or coddled-for-one-minute egg. Ours doesn't. We've taken seriously the warnings about salmonella in uncooked or even undercooked eggs. So here is our recipe, unauthentic as all get-out, but we think you'll like it. We do.

- 1 large head romaine lettuce
- 2 or 3 anchovies or a 3-inch strip of anchovy paste
- ½ teaspoon cracked black peppercorns
- ⅓ cup extra-virgin olive oil
- ¼ cup grated Parmesan cheese
- 1½ tablespoons red-wine vinegar
- 1 tablespoon freshly squeezed lemon juice
- 1 to 1½ tablespoons garlic
- 1 teaspoon dry mustard
- ½ teaspoon celery salt (optional)
- 3 dashes Tabasco sauce
- ⅓ teaspoon Worcestershire sauce

garnish:

Niçoise-style olives
Freshly grated Parmesan cheese
Grated egg white

Wash and dry the lettuce. (We like to use one of those plastic salad spinners, but Barbara's father used to meticulously dry each leaf with a dish towel.) Put in the refrigerator until ready to toss.

Into a blender or food processor with a metal blade (we prefer the former) put the anchovies or anchovy paste (you can leave out the anchovies if you really hate them, but they blend with the other ingredients and don't make the dressing taste like anchovies), peppercorns (you can crack these with a rolling pin or use a peppermill if you have one that has a setting loose enough to crack rather than grind), olive oil, Parmesan cheese, vinegar, lemon juice, garlic, dry mustard, celery salt, Tabasco sauce, and Worcestershire sauce. Blend thoroughly.

One tablespoon dressing Exchanges per serving: 1½ fat
Calories: 74 Protein: 1.5 gm Carbohydrate: 1 gm Fat: 7 gm
Fiber: 3 gm Cholesterol: 2.5 mg Sodium: 173 mg

You can either tear the leaves of romaine into pieces and toss, or leave the leaves whole and spoon the sauce over the leaves. Either way, go easy on the dressing: you don't want a puddle of Caesar soup in the bottom of the salad bowl or plate. We like to garnish the salad with a few small black Niçoise-style olives and, if you can afford the fat, some more grated Parmesan or, preferably, some Parmesan shaved from a piece. We sometimes give a nod to the traditional egg by grating some egg white into the bowl before tossing, or grating it on top of the whole-leaf salad.

We usually forgo the traditional croutons since they have extra carbohydrate and fat. June prefers to just have a crusty piece of French bread with it. One of the advantages of not having a raw or coddled egg in the dressing is that if you don't use all the dressing you can keep it in the refrigerator and use it later on without fear.

If you're absolutely forbidden any cheese at all, you can leave it out. When you do, the dressing will be strikingly similar to the dressing used on the following.

Cobb Salad

Serves 4

Cobb salad was supposedly born when there was a lack of the wherewithal for a standard chef's salad. It is basically a chopped salad of whatever greens, vegetables, and protein you happen to have on hand. We've made some wonderful unauthentic Cobb salads in just this way—and like them just as well as the more standard variety. But remember that the variations on this theme can be infinite, and if you don't have or can't find all the ingredients—especially all those different greens—just use what you do have and can find.

- ¼ head iceberg lettuce
- ½ bunch watercress
- 1 small bunch curly endive or chicory
- ¼ head romaine lettuce
- 1 tablespoon minced chives
- 1 medium tomato, peeled, seeded, and diced
- 1 cooked chicken breast
- 1½ hard-boiled eggs, diced
- 1 or 2 strips bacon (optional)
- ¼ cup Roquefort, Gorgonzola, or blue cheese (optional)

dressing:

- ¼ cup water
- ¼ cup red-wine vinegar
- ¼ teaspoon sugar equivalent of granulated fructose or artificial sweetener
- 1½ teaspoons freshly squeezed lemon juice
- ½ teaspoon salt (optional)
- ½ teaspoon black pepper, preferably freshly ground, fairly coarsely
- ¾ teaspoon English or Dijon mustard
- ½ large or 1 small clove garlic, minced
- ¼ cup extra-virgin olive oil
- ¾ cup vegetable oil

Finely chop and place in a large bowl lettuce, watercress, endive or chicory (we've sometimes used regular endive and/or fennel), romaine lettuce, chives (or, if you don't have them, green-onion tops). Place the tomato, chicken, and egg in the bowl on top of the greens.

The authentic recipe also calls for a slightly more necessary (as far as flavor is concerned) evil: bacon. Rather than using the recommended 3 strips, we use 2 (if Barbara's making it) or 1 (if June is). We wrap the strips (or strip) in paper towels and zap until crisp and dry in the microwave and crumble on top of the other salad ingredients. Another fat bearer is also supposed to be crumbled onto the salad: 1/4 cup Roquefort or Gorgonzola or blue cheese. Let your conscience—and your cholesterol—be your guide here. Chill the ingredients until serving time.

This recipe yields way more dressing than you'll need, but you might as well make a lot of it and keep it in the refrigerator to use later. Place all the ingredients in a jar (the better to shake in later). Chill the dressing. When you're ready to serve the salad, shake the shucks out of the dressing and put just enough on the salad to lightly coat the ingredients. Put in just a little at first. You can always add more, but you can't take it out. Toss the salad and serve.

4 servings using 1 tablespoon dressing per serving Exchanges per serving: 1/2 vegetable; 1 1/2 medium-fat meat; 3 fat Calories: 206 Protein: 12 gm Carbohydrate: 3 gm Fat: 15 gm Fiber: 1 gm Cholesterol: 107 mg Sodium: 325 mg

Incidentally, if you want to make this a main course and need more protein, just throw in another diced cooked chicken breast.

DINNER DISHES FROM AROUND THE WORLD: UNITED STATES

Comfort Me with Meat Loaf

Serves 4

In the chaotic modern world, many of us are turning to comfort foods, *things that make us feel warm and cozy and taken care of the way we were when we were children (if we were lucky!). One of the most popular comfort foods is meat loaf. It's even appearing on the menus of some of Los Angeles's most trendy restaurants such as 72 Market Street and Engine Company Number 28. Like most Americans, we love meat loaf. We love it hot, we love it even more cold; we love it as a main course and we love it in sandwiches. We've tried dozens of recipes over the years, and although all are delicious—it's hard to make a bad meat loaf—we've settled on this one because it's exceptionally easy, different, and tasty.*

- 2 eggs, beaten
- ½ cup finely chopped onion
- 2 tablespoons drained bottled horseradish
- 4 tablespoons rolled oats (not the instant variety)
- 1½ pounds ground chuck
- 2 tablespoons ketchup
- Salt and freshly ground pepper (optional)

Stir all the ingredients together in a bowl. (A healthy variation is to use half ground turkey and half lean chuck. When we do this we add 1 teaspoon of beef-stock-base crystals or a ground-up beef-bouillon cube to give it more flavor.) Form into two 3-by-5-inch loaves, place in a shallow baking pan, and bake at 400 degrees for half an hour. Note: if you prefer, rather than putting the ketchup into the mixture, you can put it on top just before baking. It's good either way.

4 servings Exchanges per serving: 1½ medium-fat meat
Calories: 110 Protein: 8 gm Carbohydrate: 2 gm Fat: 7 gm
Fiber: 0.26 gm Cholesterol: 54 mg Sodium: 52 mg

Mashed Potatoes with Green Onions

Serves 4

For total comfort the only thing to serve with meat loaf is mashed potatoes. In fact, mashed potatoes are the ultimate comfort dish. This healthy version, flavor-heightened with scallions, is so fast and easy that you now have no excuse to ever again use instant mashed potatoes, which are a whopping 80 on the Glycemic Index.

- 2 russet potatoes
- ⅔ cup nonfat milk
- 1 tablespoon melted butter
- ¼ cup chopped green onions

Microwave potatoes in the usual way (wash, prick with fork, wrap with a paper towel, cook between 5 and 10 minutes until they yield to a gentle squeeze; turn once halfway through the cooking period). Remove from oven, and let rest (still wrapped) for 5 minutes.

Next, in a 1-quart microwave bowl, put milk, butter, and green onions (you can also use chives) plus a little salt and pepper. Microwave uncovered at high for 2 minutes. Peel the potatoes and put them through a ricer or the medium disk of a food mill and add to the milk-and-green onion mixture. Stir well, adding a little more milk if you prefer a softer consistency.

4 servings Exchanges per serving: 2 starch; ½ fat Calories: 150 Protein: 4 gm Carbohydrate: 27 gm Fat: 3 gm Fiber: 2 gm Cholesterol: 8 mg Sodium: 58 mg

Crab (and Just About Anyfish) Cakes

Serves 6

If June ever played that game about what you would order for your last meal on earth, there's no doubt what she would select: crab cakes. She's never been known to pass one up on a menu. Not that she hasn't had some losers—greasy and with more bread crumbs than crab. But she's had some winners, too. Among those that live in the annals of her crab-cake memory are those from the Fog City Diner in San Francisco, Obrycki's in Baltimore, and (surprise!) the Hyatt Dulles just outside Washington, D.C. June likes crab cakes so much that we frequently make them at home and sometimes make them when we don't have any crab. We've made this recipe with fresh crab or canned crab or frozen crab. We've made it with half crab and half canned tuna when we didn't have enough crab on hand. We've made it with all canned tuna when that was all there was. We've made it with fresh salmon—especially when it's on sale (poaching it first in water with a slice of lemon, a few peppercorns, a clove, and some parsley). And—maybe the best way of all—we've made it with alder-smoked salmon from Oregon, available from many mail-order catalogues. We've even made it with whatever leftover fish we've brought home from restaurants in doggie bags. So here it is. Make it any way you like. Just make it!

- 1 large egg, beaten
- 1 tablespoon low-fat mayonnaise
- 4 drops Tabasco sauce
- 1 tablespoon lemon juice
- 1 teaspoon Worcestershire sauce
- 1/8 teaspoon ground cloves
- 1/2 teaspoon paprika
- 1/4 teaspoon dry mustard
- 2 tablespoons green onions, minced
- Salt and freshly ground pepper to taste
- 1 pound crab meat
- 3 tablespoons dry bread crumbs or cracker crumbs
- 2 tablespoons oil

horseradish sauce:

- 3 tablespoons low-fat mayonnaise
- 1 teaspoon drained bottled horseradish
- 1 tablespoon minced fresh parsley leaves

sherry cayenne mayonnaise:

- 3 tablespoons low-fat mayonnaise
- 1 teaspoon dry sherry
- Cayenne pepper to taste

herbal spice mayonnaise:

- 3 tablespoons low-fat mayonnaise
- 1 teaspoon (or more to taste) Arizona Herbal Spice Dip Mix

In a bowl combine egg, mayonnaise, Tabasco sauce, lemon juice, Worcestershire sauce, cloves, paprika, dry mustard, green onions, salt and freshly ground pepper to taste. Lightly but thoroughly stir in crabmeat (or whatever fish or combination of fish you will). Add dry bread crumbs or cracker crumbs. (If the mixture seems excessively moist, add just a few more crumbs.) Form into 6 patties. Keep them as light as possible; don't pack them down into dense disks. Let them rest, uncovered, on foil or wax paper for around 15 minutes.

Heat oil in a nonstick pan and sauté over medium heat until golden brown on one side; turn and do the same thing on the other side.

6 servings Exchanges per serving: 2 lean meat; 1 fat Calories: 126 Protein: 13 gm Carbohydrate: 3 gm Fat: 6 gm Fiber: 0.2 gm Cholesterol: 87 mg Sodium: 317 mg

Serve with lemon wedges or one of the following sauces. For Horseradish Sauce mix together the mayonnaise, horseradish, and parsley. For Sherry Cayenne Mayonnaise mix together the mayonnaise, dry sherry, and cayenne pepper. Or use the Herbal Spice Mayonnaise, which is particularly good on salmon cakes because it has dill in it. Mix mayonnaise and 1 teaspoon (or more to taste) of Arizona Herbal Spice Dip Mix (available from Arizona Champagne Sauces and Mustards, phone 1-800-342-9336). Make this at least a half hour prior to serving so the seasonings (which are dehydrated) can blend into the sauce.

Note: if you make fish cakes frequently, you can vary the taste by making the Maryland style (substitute 1 teaspoon Old Bay Seasoning for the other spices) or Mexican style (add 1 teaspoon minced canned green chiles—not jalapeño; they're too hot for this) or curried (add ½ teaspoon curry powder).

THE PACIFIC RIM

We feel particularly blessed to live in a Pacific Rim state. We're a Western gateway to the East as well as a gateway from the East through which pass exciting cuisines. We can try these in restaurants or, if we're lucky, go through the gateway and try them in the countries themselves and then reproduce them in our own kitchens.

INDIA

Jaqua Chicken Tandoori

Serves 8

Here's yet another Indian chicken dish; if any country has taken chicken out of the prosaic, India has. This version was given to us years ago by one of our colleagues, Los Angeles Valley College home-economics professor Ida Jaqua. It never disappoints us or our guests. It's also extremely low in fat since the skin is removed from the chicken before cooking and you grill or broil it without oil.

- 2 chickens, quartered, broilers of approximately 2½ pounds each
- 1 medium onion, chopped
- 1 pint plain nonfat yoghurt
- ½ cup fresh lime juice
- 1 teaspoon salt
- 2 teaspoons powdered ginger
- 1 teaspoon turmeric
- 1 teaspoon cumin
- 1 teaspoon coriander
- 1 teaspoon saffron threads
- ¼ teaspoon cayenne pepper
- ¼ teaspoon cinnamon
- ¼ teaspoon cloves
- ¼ teaspoon nutmeg

garnish:
Slices of onion and lime

First you skin the 2 broilers, which you have had split into quarters. Make three slashes on each piece so that the marinade can penetrate. Arrange the chicken in a single layer in a large baking pan (not aluminum).

The marinade is made in a food processor. First chop the onion and put it aside. Then put into the processor the yoghurt, lime juice, salt, ginger, and spices. Blend this with an on-and-off motion until smooth. Add the chopped onion and mix well.

Pour the marinade over the chicken, turning to coat on all sides. Cover the pan with foil or plastic wrap and place in the refrigerator for 12 to 24 hours. (We have cheated on this time recommendation and the chicken still had plenty of flavor.)

The final step is to barbecue the chicken on your grill—unless, of course, you own one of those marvelous tandoori ovens that you see in the better Indian restaurants. We have the next-best thing in our patio, a Kamado-Hibachi Pot—an earthenware oven made by an ancient Japanese process.

Remove the chicken from the refrigerator 30 minutes before cooking. Place pieces on an oiled barbecue grill or under your oven broiler rack and cook 12 to 15 minutes on each side. To test for doneness, pierce the thickest part with a knife point. Escaping juices should be yellow, with no trace of pink.

Arrange the chicken pieces on a large platter in an attractive pattern. Garnish with onion and lime.

8 servings Exchanges per serving: 3 lean meat; 1/4 skim milk
Calories: 154 Protein: 27 gm Carbohydrate: 3 gm Fat: 4 gm
Fiber: 0 gm Cholesterol: 115 mg Sodium: 138 mg

You can serve your tandoori chicken with basmati rice, which has a nice perfumy flavor. But if that's not available in your area, Dr. Brown's recipe is a good and exotic alternative.

Dr. Brown's Wild and Brown Rice Pilaf

Serves 4

- ½ cup raw wild rice
- ½ cup raw short-grain brown rice
- 2½ cups chicken stock
- 2 tablespoons minced parsley
- 1 cup coarsely chopped mushrooms
- Freshly ground pepper
- 4 tablespoons lightly toasted almond slivers

Combine in a medium-size saucepan: wild rice, brown rice, stock, parsley, mushrooms, and pepper to taste. Cover, bring to a boil, and simmer for 1 hour. During the last 5 minutes, stir in almond slivers. Makes approximately 2 cups.

4 servings Exchanges per serving: 1 starch; 1 fat Calories: 149
Protein: 5 gm Carbohydrate: 24 gm Fat: 4 gm Fiber: 3 gm
Cholesterol: 0 mg Sodium: 501 mg

To round out your Indian feast, here's a vegetable recipe we picked up in Sri Lanka. It's named not after the detective in the raincoat, but after the capital city.

Spinach Colombo

Serves 2

- 1 tablespoon vegetable oil
- 1 medium onion, minced
- 1½ teaspoons cumin
- ¾ teaspoon powdered coriander
- 1 large bunch chopped spinach
- 2 chopped tomatoes

In a large skillet or wok, heat oil and slowly cook onion until soft. Add cumin and coriander. Stir until mixed with the onion. Increase heat and add spinach a little at a time, stirring constantly. When all the spinach has been added, add tomatoes (slice across the equator and squeeze out the juice and seeds before chopping). Cook uncovered, stirring occasionally, for 3 minutes.

2 servings Exchanges per serving: 1½ fat; 2 vegetable Calories: 115
Protein: 3 gm Carbohydrate: 11 gm Fat: 7 gm Fiber: 4 gm
Cholesterol: 0 mg Sodium: 57 mg

CHINA

Dim Sum

We'll start our cooking adventures in China—the way they sometimes start the eating adventures in midmorning—with dim sum (also sometimes spelled *deem sum* because it's pronounced that way). Dim sum seems to gain a lot of meanings in the translation. We've read it as "heart's delight," "little jewels that tug at the heart," "heart warmers," and "little heart."

We first encountered dim sum in Japan, when we were at lunch in a Chinese restaurant. Women were pushing steam trays and carts around the room, and people were selecting dishes from them and eating happily. We couldn't order any because we didn't know what was in them (we spoke neither Japanese nor Chinese). Later research revealed that dim sum were varied items such as deep-fried egg rolls, yeast buns filled with vegetables or meat, various ingredients in thin dough, plus some things too unusual to describe.

To be honest, June doesn't like going to dim sum restaurants because she has trouble calculating her meal, especially in cases when she has no idea what she's eating (it could be a disguised chicken foot). Barbara, of course, loves dim sum restaurants.

Now we usually compromise and create them at home. It's not hard to do, but it is a bit time-consuming.

What we suggest is to make a whole lot at once and freeze the ones you don't use; then later, when you take them out, you have an effortless treat. Also, rather than eating a whole pile of dim sum for a meal, we use a couple of them for appetizers and then follow up with a stir-fry dish such as the Crab in Black-Bean Sauce we tell about later. Sometimes the wonton coverings and the vegetables in the meal provide enough carbohydrate so you don't need to have a separate serving of rice, or else just a very small one (4 wonton wrappers are 1 Starch/Bread Exchange).

Mainly Shrimp Siu Mai

Makes 24 siu mai

This is sometimes spelled shu mai *(again because that's how it's pronounced).* Siu mai *are little pouches of good stuff—sometimes pork, sometimes shrimp, sometimes a combination of those. Here's one of our favorites.*

Happily, with the internationalization of America you can probably find wonton skins in your market. They're a real drag to make because you have to make them so thin, and thin is important in wonton skins—especially for diabetics.

- 1 pound raw shrimp
- 6 dried Chinese mushrooms
- 6 water chestnuts (canned)
- 3 tablespoons bamboo shoots (canned)
- 3 green onions
- 8 ounces lean pork, minced very fine
- 1 tablespoon low sodium soy sauce
- 1 tablespoon dry sherry
- 1 teaspoon sesame oil
- 1 egg white, beaten
- 24 wonton wrappers

For the *siu mai* filling, clean the shrimp, removing the shell and cutting down the outside rounded part to remove the black vein. (A special shrimp knife helps a lot here.) If your shrimp are tiny, keep out 24 of them; if they're medium, keep out 12; if they're pretty big, keep out 8. If they're *huge,* keep out 6. Chop the rest of the shrimp.

Soak the Chinese mushrooms in hot water for a half hour. Remove and throw away the stems and chop the caps into small pieces. Also chop the water chestnuts, bamboo shoots, and the green onions. Mince the pork. Combine all the chopped and minced ingredients in a bowl. Add the soy sauce, sherry, sesame oil, and beaten egg white. Mix well. Now the fun begins.

Take a wonton wrapper and place either in the palm of your hand or in the circle made by joining your thumb and index finger. Place a heaping teaspoon of the filling in the center of the wonton skin, and gather the sides up around the filling in pleats so that it looks like a little money bag. There will be an open space at the top into which you will insert a tiny shrimp (or ½, ⅓, or ¼ of a larger one). Put the filled wrappers into a pan or bowl and cover with a damp towel. Proceed until you've made 24 *siu mai.* Put the ones you're using for that meal into a steamer, which has been lightly oiled. Cover and steam for 20 to 30 minutes. Serve either hot or cold, with dipping sauces (see below).

4 siu mai Exchanges per serving: 2 medium-fat meat; 1 starch; ½ vegetable Calories: 276 Protein: 31 gm Carbohydrate: 23 gm Fat: 5 gm Fiber: 2 gm Cholesterol: 164 mg Sodium: 212 mg

Potstickers

Makes 24 potstickers

Another variety of little hearts *we like to make are potstickers.*

- 24 wonton skins
- ¾ pound beef or pork, finely minced or ground
- 1 pound Chinese celery cabbage
- 1½ teaspoons low sodium soy sauce
- ½ teaspoon sugar equivalent of fructose or artificial sweetener
- 1 teaspoon vegetable oil
- 1 egg white

to cook:

- 1 tablespoon vegetable oil
- ½ cup water

Mince the Chinese celery cabbage (or savoy cabbage or, in desperation, regular cabbage), sprinkle with salt, wrap in a cloth or dish towel, and squeeze out as much of the liquid as you can. Combine in a bowl the finely minced beef or pork, the cabbage, the soy sauce, the fructose or artificial sweetener, and the vegetable oil (if you like the taste of sesame oil, use that).

Lightly beat the egg white. Use a Joyce Chen plastic "Dumplings Plus" press or the one made by the Frugal Gourmet or a generic equivalent. Place the wonton skin over the dumpling press, put a teaspoon of filling in the middle, brush the outer edges with egg white (to make them stick), close the dumpling maker firmly, and remove the potsticker, putting it on a board or plate covered with a damp towel. If you don't have a dumpling maker you can just put the filling into the middle of the wonton skin, brush the edges with egg white, and press around the edges with a fork. Continue making potstickers until you've used up all the filling. Freeze the potstickers you aren't going to use at once.

Put 1 tablespoon of vegetable oil in an 8- or 9-inch *non-stick* frying pan that has a lid. We emphasize nonstick because the first time we made these, we used a regular frying pan and learned the true meaning of the term *potsticker.* Heat the oil over a medium flame and arrange the potstickers in a circle; they can touch one another. Add ½ cup water to the pan, cover, and cook over medium heat until the water has evaporated.

This should take around 6 or 7 minutes. Turn the heat down to low and continue cooking with the lid still on for another 2 or 3 minutes, or until the dumplings are golden brown (but not burned!) on the bottom. Gently loosen the potstickers with a spatula, remove carefully, and place the potstickers *browned side up* on a platter or on individual dishes. Serve hot, with a selection of dipping sauces.

4 potstickers Exchanges per serving: 2 medium-fat meat; 1 starch; 1 vegetable Calories: 260 Protein: 16 gm Carbohydrate: 26 gm Fat: 9 gm Fiber: 1.6 gm Cholesterol: 33 mg Sodium: 120 mg

Dipping Sauces

Use a selection of these sauces with both *siu mai* and potstickers.

Mustard. This is June's favorite. We've tried various brands of Chinese mustard, both prepared and dry, but the best we've come up with is Coleman's dry mustard mixed with milk. Even when you use nonfat as we always do, it makes for a very creamy (and hot!) product, and it's diabetically free. Be careful not to add too much milk or it becomes so thin that it runs into the other sauces on your plate.

Chinese rice-wine vinegar. This is another freebie, but be sure to use the mild variety.

Chile oil. Barbara's favorite. Available in major supermarkets or Asian specialty markets. Also diabetically free, especially since you don't dare use more than a few drops.

Soy sauce (if you can take the extra sodium). Use it either straight or with minced ginger or garlic.

Plum sauce and/or hoisin sauce. These are full of sugar and are to be used only to indulge the civilians in your dining group.

Dr. Brown's Chinese Chicken Salad

Serves 4

Chinese chicken salad is a popular favorite on Southern California menus. This version, by our friend Dr. Ron Brown, is particularly good and particularly healthy.

- 2 cups shredded cooked chicken
- ½ cup raw carrots
- ½ cup Chinese pea pods or sugar snap peas
- 8 ounces sliced water chestnuts (canned)
- ½ bunch cilantro (optional)
- 1 cup raw bean sprouts
- 3 green onions, chopped
- 5 cups shredded lettuce
- 1 tablespoon toasted sesame seeds
- 2 tablespoons chopped walnuts

dressing:

- 3 tablespoons rice wine vinegar
- 2 tablespoons sesame oil (dark, if possible)
- 2 or 3 drops Tabasco sauce
- ½ teaspoon salt (optional)
- Ground pepper to taste
- ½ packet Equal

Make the dressing by combining the rice vinegar (or white-wine vinegar), sesame oil, a few drops Tabasco, the salt (optional), and ground pepper to taste, and ½ packet Equal.

Mix half the dressing in a large bowl with the cooked chicken. Let marinate while you prepare the vegetables: toss together the carrots (cut into matchstick size), the pea pods, water chestnuts, cilantro (optional), bean sprouts, green onions, and lettuce (the greener, the more nutritious). Toss with the chicken and the remainder of the dressing. Mix in sesame seeds and walnuts.

4 servings Exchanges per serving: 2 lean meat; 2 fat; 3 vegetable
Calories: 338 Protein: 29 gm Carbohydrate: 19 gm Fat: 17 gm
Fiber: 5 gm Cholesterol: 75 mg Sodium: 357 mg

Woking your way to health. Wok cooking or stir-frying is healthy because you cook in such a very small amount of oil. And since you cook so fast and since most of the water or stock you cook in is evaporated or incorporated into the sauce, the vitamins and minerals are retained. It's also healthy because it takes so little time to do (once you've prepared the ingredients) that when you're in a hurry you're more likely to cook up something for yourself than resort to fast food or commercial frozen dinners.

For the best wok, buy a cheap steel one at least 12 inches in diameter. These are available in Asian markets. Don't buy a fancy electric one, because they heat up slowly and cannot be turned down quickly. If you don't already have a lid big enough to cover the wok, buy one. You'll also need a long-handled, scooplike stirrer with the bottom curved to match the shape of the wok. This is the standard wok tool used to shovel ingredients up and away from the hot spot in the bottom.

To cure your cheapie wok, if it has the usual lacquer coating, fill it with water, add 1 tablespoon baking soda, and boil for 15 to 20 minutes. Then it's easy to remove the coating with a plastic scouring pad. Dry the wok over low heat, and while it's hot, rub it with a paper towel moistened with vegetable oil.

After you use the wok, always soak it in hot water with detergent, scrub with a sponge or kitchen brush (never steel wool!), rinse, gently heat dry, and rub down with an oiled paper towel.

Over the months as you use your wok, it will start to turn black. Do not fret and do not clean the black off. For a wok, black is beautiful. It means it's well cured and better to cook in.

Although stir-frying comes to us from China, it can be used for any kind of cuisine. An excellent introductory book, *The Sunset Stir-Fry Cookbook*, has such non-Chinese recipes as Huevos Revueltos Rancheros, Pork Tenderloin Normandy, and Italian Stir-Fried Pasta.

Stir-Frying Vegetables

To stir-fry fresh vegetables, simply prepare them by cutting them into small, uniform pieces or slices (so they cook fast and are all done at the same time). Then place the wok over high heat and add (for 2 cups of vegetables) ½ tablespoon of oil (preferably canola, avocado, or peanut). When the oil is hot put in all of the vegetables at once and stir for all you're worth for 1 minute. Add two tablespoons of water or chicken stock or beef broth. Slap on the lid and cook for about 3 to 5 minutes; we can't tell you exactly how long to cook because some kinds of vegetables cook faster than others and we don't know how well cooked you like your vegetables. Some trendy restaurants in Los Angeles serve their vegetables so raw they seem to be only barely heated. (These are the same ones that prefer fish to have a cool uncooked center because they have a deathly fear of drying it out.) You'll need to experiment to see what you and yours prefer. You can combine vegetables by either putting the ones that take less cooking time in later or by cooking them separately and then combining them at the end for a quick hot-hit.

If you double the amount of vegetables, double the amount of oil and liquid, but keep the cooking time the same.

To give your vegetables a Chinese taste, stir minced garlic and/or minced ginger into the oil before you add the vegetables, and add low-sodium soy sauce for half the liquid. To make the thicker sauce that you find in Chinese restaurants, instead of adding soy sauce and liquid and covering, make a mixture of ½ tablespoon cornstarch, ½ tablespoon water, ½ tablespoon low-sodium soy sauce, and ½ cup chicken broth. After stir-frying the vegetables, add this mixture and keep stirring until the sauce boils and becomes thick. But be careful not to cook it until it's dry and pasty.

Crab in Black-Bean Sauce

Serves 4

When crab is on sale we usually make this dish. We particularly love it because you get down and dirty, eating with both your hands and licking your fingers. Also, since you're cracking the shells and picking out every last morsel of the sweet meat, you eat slowly, taking lots of time, and you have great feelings of satisfaction, although you're not eating all that much. (That's why we think eating artichokes is good for diabetics!)

1 2-pound crab (or 2 one-pound ones)
1½ tablespoons canned salted black beans
1 large or 2 small cloves garlic
1 teaspoon minced fresh ginger
¼ pound lean pork (optional)

for the sauce:
1 tablespoon cornstarch
1 tablespoon low-sodium soy sauce
1 tablespoon dry sherry
½ cup chicken stock
1 egg, lightly beaten
3 green onions, chopped

to cook:
3 tablespoons oil

Preparing the crab. The best way to prepare the crab is to have the butcher or fish-counter person clean and crack your crab for you. If he or she lacks the skill or time, you can do it yourself. (It's always good to learn a new kitchen skill, and once you've learned this one, besides making this more complex dish you can have a lovely simple meal of cracked crab served with lemon wedges, low-fat mayonnaise, and horseradish. But skip the cocktail sauce since that usually has sugar in it.)

Take the cooked crab and remove the top shell by grasping it and prying it off—it's not that difficult to do. You will see the gills, a kind of fingery fibrous material. Remove these with a sharp knife. Wash out all the rest of the stuff inside that can be washed out. Break off the claws and crack them with a hammer or mallet. Cut the body down the middle and then cut each half into three pieces, leaving the legs attached.

Rinse and drain the black beans (available in the Oriental-foods section of markets). Mash the beans and combine with the garlic (finely minced or put through a press) and the ginger.

to this mixture add the pork. (The pork is optional but gives a little extra protein, which may be needed in the diabetic diet.)

Prepare a sauce using the cornstarch, soy sauce, dry sherry (or Chinese wine, and lots of luck in finding it), and chicken stock. In another bowl combine the egg with the green onions.

Heat the wok and, when it is hot, add 3 tablespoons oil (peanut oil gives a distinctive Oriental taste, but avocado or canola are okay, too). When the oil is hot, add the pork and garlic-ginger mixture. Stir-fry briskly for about 2 minutes. Add the crab and stir-fry for another couple of minutes.

Add the cornstarch/soy/wine/chicken-stock sauce and keep stirring until the sauce boils and starts to thicken. Add the egg and green onions and stir-fry for about half a minute, or until the egg just starts to set. Serve instantly (have the guests waiting), with rice (white or brown as you prefer).

4 servings   Exchanges per serving: 4 medium-fat meat; ½ starch
Calories: 287   Protein: 26 gm   Carbohydrate: 9 gm   Fat: 15 gm
Fiber: 1.4 gm   Cholesterol: 159 mg   Sodium: 454 mg

Now we'll change directions and head east to the West, first touching down for some samples of our original favorite cuisine and one we still love, although in a different way than before.

FRANCE

French cooking has been somewhat out of favor in this country for a few years. People no longer want the rich sauces that it was famous for, and the lighter *cuisine minceur* never really caught on. But something good is happening to French cooking. French bistros are starting to pop up, and people (including us) really like the simpler peasant fare—and the lower prices. Here are a few favorite bistro-style recipes.

Céleri Rémoulade

Serves 4

This is a classic and very satisfying French vegetable hors d'oeuvre that we've seldom seen in a restaurant or deli here. You can either go to France for it (try it at Scossa on the Place Victor Hugo in Paris) or make it yourself (it's no trouble). The only little obstacle is that its basic ingredient, celery root (celeriac), is usually available only in large markets, and it does take a food shredder or processor that can cut it into strips about one-eighth-inch wide.

1 large celery root

for the dressing:
½ teaspoon Dijon mustard
2 tablespoons wine vinegar
⅓ cup salad oil

or:
⅓ cup low-fat mayonnaise
½ teaspoon Dijon mustard

serve with:
Fresh chopped parsley

Pare off the fibrous outside of the celery root. Wash off any remaining dirt, and then cut it into chunks and shred it. Take your choice of dressings: (1) Dijon mustard beaten together with wine vinegar and salad oil; or (2) mayonnaise mixed with Dijon mustard. Mix the shredded celery root with as much of the dressing as your diet allows and chill. Serve with fresh chopped parsley sprinkled over the top. This makes a nice first course to serve with one of the following main courses.

4 servings Exchanges per serving: 2 fat; 1 vegetable Calories: 106 Protein: 5 gm Carbohydrate: 3 gm Fat: 10 gm Fiber: 1 gm Cholesterol: 0 mg Sodium: 60 mg

Ragoût d'Agneau à la Française, AKA Lamb Stew

Serves 6

It must be true that simple pleasures are the best, for we've found that guests slosh compliments all over the table when we serve this simple lamb stew.

- 3 tablespoons olive or salad oil
- 2 pounds lean lamb
- 1 chopped onion
- 1 clove garlic
- 1 tablespoon flour
- 1½ cups chicken broth
- 1 crushed bay leaf
- 1 pinch marjoram
- ½ cup dry white wine
- Salt and pepper to taste
- 8 small white onions, peeled
- 3 sliced carrots
- 3 medium potatoes, peeled and cut into chunks

serve with:
- Fresh chopped parsley
- French bread

Heat oil in a large pot. Add the lamb cut into one-inch cubes. Often it's best to take the easy way out and use leg of lamb. Brown the lamb over a brisk flame; then take it out of the pan and set it aside. In about 1 tablespoon oil that you've left in the pot sauté the onion and garlic (that you've put through a garlic press) until transparent and gold. Put the lamb back into the pot and sprinkle the flour over all. Pour in the chicken broth, add the bay leaf, a fat pinch of marjoram, the white wine, and salt and pepper to taste. Stir everything well, put the lid on the pot, and simmer 30 to 35 minutes. Every once in a while skim off with a tablespoon any fat that may have accumulated on top.

At the end of this first cooking period, add the onions, and let the pot continue to bubble lightly for another quarter of an hour. Throw in the carrots and the potatoes. Continue cooking at the same slow rate for about another half hour, or until the vegetables are tender but not mushy. When you serve the stew, dust each portion generously with chopped fresh parsley.

Serve the stew with French bread with which to sop up the lovely juices. (To heat French bread, wet your hands, then dry them on your uncut loaf of bread and put it in a hot oven until the crust is crisp.)

6 servings Exchanges per serving: 4 medium-fat meat; 1½ fat; 1 starch; 1 vegetable Calories: 496 Protein: 47 gm Carbohydrate: 28 gm Fat: 19 gm Fiber: 4 gm Cholesterol: 135 mg Sodium: 318 mg

You don't need much else with this stew. Start the meal with a salad or the céleri rémoulade and end it with fruit.

Roast Chicken

Serves 6

This is the classic French bistro dish—with a difference. Select a nice plump roasting chicken. A free-range chicken is the best if you can find it, but if not, try to get a chicken that has at least been grown in your state or very close by. Avoid chickens that have been shipped from Alabama or Arkansas (unless you live in Alabama or Arkansas) and possibly have been sitting for a few days on a railroad siding.

- 1 roasting chicken, about 4 pounds
- 5 large cloves garlic, minced
- ½ cup minced parsley
- ½ cup fresh herbs (thyme, basil, marjoram, oregano, and so on) or ¼ cup dried herbs
- Vegetable oil
- 1 lemon

for basting:

- Dry white wine or dry vermouth

Mince the garlic and combine with the parsley and the fresh herbs (thyme, basil, marjoram, oregano, and so on) or the dried herbs. Sometimes you can find mixtures of Provençal herbs in gourmet shops, and those work very well. Once we gave the recipe an Italian touch by stuffing the chicken with a combination of minced garlic, chopped fresh basil, and chopped pine nuts.

Preheat the oven to 450 degrees. Take the whole chicken in your bare hands and stuff the garlic mixture under the skin wherever you can. Stuff down from the neck and up from the nether regions—going clear up into the skin under the thighs and legs. (Yes, it *can* be done!) Wipe your hands on the chicken: you don't want to waste any of that lovely garlic mixture. Give the chicken a light vegetable-oil rubdown. Put the whole lemon into the cavity. Put the chicken into a roasting pan.

Turn the oven temperature down to 350 degrees, put the chicken in, and cook it about 20 minutes per pound. Baste it every 15 or 20 minutes with dry white wine or vermouth. It's done when the juices run clear when you stick a fork into what June calls "the hip." You'll find you've never had a more succulent, flavorful chicken, and the garlic turns quite sweet-tasting in the cooking.

6 servings Exchanges per serving: 5½ lean meat Calories: 309
Protein: 44 gm Carbohydrate: 5 gm Fat: 11 gm Fiber: 1.3 gm
Cholesterol: 134 mg Sodium: 135 mg

Another way to roast chicken for lovers of the "stinking rose" is to put 40 cloves of garlic (sometimes we've cheated and used only 25) into the cavity and roast it as above. The sweet garlic can be spread on French bread for a special treat, or you can slice it onto whatever vegetable you're serving (broccoli is particularly good) or chop it into mashed potatoes.

Once Barbara was asked what she thought of roasting a chicken with both the minced garlic under the skin and the 40 cloves in the cavity. She said she thought that would be perfect for a Halloween dinner since it would drive away any vampires that might be cruising the neighborhood.

Potatoes with a Hemingway Heart

Serves 6

The classic French accompaniment for the classic French roast chicken would be French fried potatoes. In a fat-conscious world, however, deep-frying is out. We've tried lower-fat oven-fried compromises and found that they just didn't do the job—especially one that involved dipping the potatoes in beaten egg whites.

The better way to go, we think, is to try something different, something that also adds another classic French touch—leeks. (Many moons ago, we heard Dorothy Parker speak at a library conference where she told the audience that during one period when Hemingway was living in France, he lived for six months on nothing but leeks. She then peered over her spectacles at the audience and added, "That's spelled l-e-e-k-s.") Since occasionally Hemingway might have been able to also afford a couple of potatoes, we've called this dish Potatoes with a Hemingway Heart.

1 pound leeks
3½ tablespoons plus 2 teaspoons vegetable oil *in all*
¼ cup chicken stock
⅓ cup milk
2 russet potatoes

Split the leeks lengthwise and wash thoroughly to get any dirt or grit out. Slice the white part and about an inch of the green crossways into very thin slices. (You can do this by hand or in a food processor.) Heat 1½ tablespoons of the vegetable oil in a saucepan over medium heat, add the leeks, and sauté, stirring constantly, for 2 to 3 minutes (don't let them brown). Add the chicken stock, cover, and cook for 15 to 20 minutes, or until tender. (Check occasionally to make sure the leeks aren't getting dry.) Add the milk and cook, uncovered, until the liquid is reduced and thickened. Let cool. (The dish can be prepared in advance up to this point and kept cool in the refrigerator.)

Peel the potatoes and shred by hand or with the medium shredding disk of the food processor. Immediately plunge the potatoes into enough ice water to cover for 15 minutes. Drain thoroughly in a strainer or sieve and put the potatoes in the center of a dish towel. Roll up and twist the towel, wringing out every bit of water you can.

In a large, nonstick skillet with a tight-fitting lid, heat 2 tablespoons of the vegetable oil over a medium flame. Spread half the potatoes evenly over the bottom of the skillet, smoothing and pressing them gently with the back of a spoon. Spread the leek mixture evenly over the potatoes up to ½ inch of the edge. Spread the rest of the potatoes over the top, trying not to let any leeks show through. Press down gently, making a round cake about 10 inches in diameter. Cover and cook over medium heat. (Shake the pan occasionally to make sure the potatoes are not sticking). After about 5 minutes, take off the lid to let out the steam. Dry the inside of the lid with a towel. Cover and cook (shaking occasionally) another 5 minutes. Take off the lid (again wipe it dry) and check to see if the potatoes are golden brown on the bottom. If they aren't, cook a little longer.

Now here comes the tricky part, though it's not as tricky as it sounds. Put the lid on the pan and turn the pan upside down, letting the cake drop into the lid. If the pan is totally dry, put in the remaining 2 teaspoons of oil and stir it around until the surface is lightly coated. Slide the potato cake off the lid into the pan. (The brown crispy bottom is now on top.) Cook uncovered over medium-low heat until the new bottom is golden brown. Sprinkle with parsley and, since it's so pretty, serve it on a platter, cutting individual portions at the table.

6 servings Exchanges per serving: 1 starch; 1 fat; 1 vegetable
Calories: 182 Protein: 2.5 gm Carbohydrate: 23 gm
Fat: 10 gm Fiber: 3 gm Cholesterol: 0 mg Sodium: 56 mg

This is a remarkably versatile dish. Once we didn't have any leeks so we used braised fennel. It was equally good. It would work with braised onions as well. If you have nothing to put in the middle, then put nothing in the middle and you'll have the famous Swiss potato dish Rösti.

Now we need a vegetable dish for our bistro meal—an easy one that can be made ahead of time. We need something like . . .

Martha's Ratatouille

Serves 6

Martha Kuljian, a librarian friend of ours, once served us this vegetable dish of southern France. We instantly requested the recipe and have been making it ever since; you will, too, once you've tasted it.

- 2 tablespoons olive oil
- 1 tablespoon salt (optional)
- 1 garlic clove, crushed
- 1 medium eggplant
- 4 medium zucchini
- 1 bell pepper
- 2 onions
- 2 teaspoons capers
- 1 large can Italian plum tomatoes
- Parsley

In Martha's very own words: "I use a 9-by-12-inch baking pan and line it with foil. Put the olive oil, salt (feel free to use 1 teaspoon or none), and crushed garlic in the bottom. Cut the eggplant into large pieces (2 inches or so) and toss in the oil. Cut the zucchini into ¼-inch slices, the pepper into large pieces, and the onions into eighths, I guess—anyway, into recognizable pieces. Add to pan along with the capers (I buy mine from an Italian deli in bulk), and on top put the tomatoes. I don't use the juice at all; just cut each tomato into halves or quarters, depending on size. Fresh ones are great, too. Sprinkle with parsley, preferably fresh. Cover with foil and bake at 350 degrees for 1 hour or longer, until the onion is done. I always make this at least one day ahead. [Unlike Martha, we have been known to eat it right out of the oven.] It also is delicious cold or at room temperature, with a couple of teaspoons of balsamic vinegar added, and served on a lettuce leaf."

6 servings Exchanges per serving: 1 fat; 1 vegetable Calories: 80
Protein: 2 gm Carbohydrate: 9 gm Fat: 5 gm Fiber: 3 gm
Cholesterol: 0.8 mg Sodium: 1074 mg (with 1 tablespoon salt)

Shrimp au Pernod

Serves 4

This is a nice celebratory dish, because you can dazzle your guests—or yourself—by igniting the Pernod at the table. It's served at Los Angeles's historic Biltmore Hotel. Pernod, incidentally, is a yellow-colored, anise-flavored French aperitif. Barbara traditionally has a small glass of it her first night in Paris. (You fill the glass with water and the liquid becomes milky white.) You probably won't want to invest in a big bottle of Pernod. Just get one of those bottles like the ones they serve on airlines, and you'll have plenty to make the dish three or four times.

- 2 tablespoons extra-virgin olive oil
- 3 to 4 tablespoons shallots, finely chopped
- 1 teaspoon chopped garlic
- 1 teaspoon chopped parsley
- 16 jumbo shrimp, peeled and deveined
- 2 tablespoons Pernod
- Salt (optional), pepper, and cayenne

Heat the olive oil in a skillet over medium heat. In the oil sauté the shallots, garlic, and parsley. To this add the shrimp and sauté until pink. Add the Pernod and ignite. (It lights more reliably if you warm it before adding.) Now season with a little salt (optional), pepper, and cayenne. *Voilà!* It's ready.

4 servings Exchanges per serving: 2 lean meat; 1½ fat
Calories: 133 Protein: 6 gm Carbohydrate: 6 gm Fat: 7 gm
Fiber: 0.1 gm Cholesterol: 43 mg Sodium: 44 mg

Couscous

Serves 4

Couscous is a good accompaniment for your shrimp dish and many other dishes as well. This quick, easy-to-prepare, and versatile product comes to France—and to us—via Morocco. Since it's made of hard durum wheat (as the best pastas are), you might call it a kind of granular pasta. The raisins are optional if you don't have the Fruit Exchange available or prefer to save it for your dessert.

- ¼ cup raisins (optional)
- 1 tablespoon butter, margarine, or avocado oil
- ½ cup finely chopped onion
- 1½ cups boiling water
- 2 teaspoons lemon juice
- ¼ teaspoon ground cumin
- 1 cup couscous
- Salt to taste (optional)

Cover the raisins with lukewarm water for 15 to 20 minutes; drain and reserve for later use. Melt the butter, margarine, or oil in a saucepan and add the onion. Cook, stirring, over low heat until the onion is limp but not brown. Add the boiling water, lemon juice, ground cumin, and the raisins. Bring to a boil, remove from the heat, and add the couscous. Add salt to taste (optional). Immediately clap on the lid and let stand for 5 minutes. Uncover, fluff with a fork, and serve.

4 servings Exchanges per serving: 1 starch; ½ fat Calories: 108
Protein: 2 gm Carbohydrate: 19 gm Fat: 3 gm Fiber: 2 gm
Cholesterol: 8 mg Sodium: 35 mg

ITALY

Ah, home again, in Italy. We have such an affinity for Italian food these days that we're beginning to feel that in some previous incarnation we must have dwelt along the Arno or beside Lake Como or in a town clinging to a cliff above the Mediterranean. And it seems that most Americans share our passion for Italian cuisine. In survey after survey, Italian restaurants lead the list as the favorite place to dine. And Italian cuisine is healthy, what with its use of the monounsaturate olive oil and its emphasis on vegetables and pasta (which, for some wonderful reason, doesn't raise a diabetic's blood sugar as much as corresponding amounts of other complex-carbohydrate dishes).

Italian cooking is also easy to do. As Biba Caggiano, owner and chef of one of Sacramento's best restaurants and author of *Northern Italian Cooking,* says, "Italian food is simply outstanding and outstandingly simple."

Getting involved with Italian cooking means, when you come home after a hard day, never having to resort to fast foods or going out to a restaurant in desperation. With a freezer containing a few balls of pizza dough, a bag of ravioli, and some containers of homemade tomato sauce and a cupboard containing pastas of various kinds, a bag of Arborio rice, some dried mushrooms, and bottles of extra-virgin olive oil and balsamic vinegar, you always have the makings of a healthy, easy-to-prepare dinner that you and your family will relish.

Pizza from Hell (It's Heavenly!)

Makes 4 8″–9″ pizzas

You can say about pizza what was once said about another pervasive element in society—you guess which: when it's good it's terrific, and even when it's not too great, it's still pretty good. To our minds and taste buds, pizza moved into the realm of terrific in a dark, cavernous restaurant called Inferno ("hell") in Madonna di Campiglio, an isolated ski resort in Italy. There we first experienced pizza made in an appropriately "hot as hell" wood-fired brick oven. Contrary to the restaurant's name, its pizza was pure heaven. June found she could eat twice as many slices of these crisp, thin-crusted disks of delight without going over her carbohydrate allotment as she could the pizza we were accustomed to back home. The toppings were much more interesting and generally more healthy than the fat-laden cheese-and-sausage-and-pepperoni variety usually available to us.

Once we returned home we often longed for such pizza. Our dreams came true when Alice Waters, of Chez Panisse in Berkeley, opened a café upstairs from the restaurant and began serving amazing pizza. The next time we went to the Bay Area, we went to the Chez Panisse café and had what was like the Pizza from Hell in Madonna di Campiglio: the product of a wood-fired brick oven, with a light and crispy crust and interesting toppings.

Not long after that, Wolfgang Puck put Los Angeles on the pizza map with his place on the Sunset Strip, Spago, where Hollywood movers and shakers made reservations a month in advance to try—among other culinary wonders—his duck-sausage pizza and later on down the line his smoked-salmon pizza.

The reason we're carrying on at such great length about pizza is that we want to inspire you to do as we now do—make an ever-changing panoply of Pizzas from Hell in your own kitchen. You'll find that the pizza you make is a hundred times better than what you've tried in the pizza chains and a thousand times more appropriate to the diabetic diet. You'll thrill and delight your friends.

To make Pizza from Hell, you will need to get a few tools of the trade: a peel (the large wooden paddle used to put the pizza in the oven and take it out; available by mail order from Williams-Sonoma, phone 1-800-541-2233; or from Sassafras, 1-800-537-4941) and a pizza stone or tiles (stones are also available from Sassafras; Salday Products has tiles set in a metal frame; 1-800-536-4941).

for the yeast mixture:

- 1 package dry yeast
- 1/4 cup warm water
- 1/2 teaspoon honey or brown sugar
- 2 tablespoons olive oil
- 1 teaspoon honey or brown sugar
- 3 cups all-purpose flour

for the dough:

- 3/4 cup water
- 1 teaspoon salt

to coat the dough:

- 1 or 2 teaspoons of olive oil

Once you're well equipped, first make your dough. Dissolve the package of dry yeast in the warm water to which you've added either the honey or brown sugar. Remain calm. This little bit of honey or brown sugar won't hurt you; it's just to get the yeast working. Let it roil around for about 10 minutes.

In another mixing bowl combine the water for the dough with the salt, olive oil, and honey or brown sugar. (Again don't worry; most of this dissipates in the cooking.)

Put the flour in the bowl of a food processor, which you've fitted with a metal blade. (If you don't own a food processor, you can do this in a mixing bowl, using a spoon.) With the processor running, pour the water-salt-honey-oil mixture in through the tube. When this is all mixed in, pour in the dissolved yeast. Keep the processor running until the dough forms a smooth ball. If it's sticky, put in a little more flour.

On a *very* lightly floured board (only enough flour to keep the dough from sticking) knead the dough until it is smooth and shiny and elastic. This will take around 10 minutes. Then put a teaspoon or two of olive oil into a large bowl. Roll the ball of dough around in the oil until all the surface is coated. (You don't want a crust to form on the dough.) Cover the bowl with a dish towel and let rest in a warm place until the dough rises to about double in size.

Form the dough into a cylinder and divide it into four equal parts. Form each part into a ball and put it in a sealable plastic bag. Put the bags of dough into the refrigerator, where it will keep for up to two days. (You can freeze any dough you don't want to use right away. The morning of the day you plan to use frozen dough, take it out of the freezer and put it in the refrigerator to defrost.)

About a half hour before you intend to form your pizzas, place your pizza stone or tile on the lowest shelf of your oven. Turn the oven on as high as it will go and let it heat up for the half hour.

Before you start forming your pizzas, you should have your peel ready and lightly dusted with flour or cornmeal. Take a ball of dough that you've brought to room temperature, and on a lightly floured board roll it out until it's around 6 inches in diameter. Then stretch it until its diameter increases to about 8 or 9 inches. You can do this in one of three ways. (We once sat at the counter of Postrio, Wolfgang Puck's San Francisco outpost, and watched the pizza makers in action.) If you're a beginner you can either (1) pinch and stretch your way around the pizza with thumbs and index fingers (thumbs on one side, index fingers on the other; the pizza also stretches itself a little as it hangs down) or (2) rest the pizza on your two doubled-up fists and stretch it by moving your fists apart; keep working in a circular motion. Gravity helps the stretching in this method, too.

The pros put the dough on their doubled-up fists as in method 2 and then spin it into the air—the higher, the more pro—several times until it's the desired size. Barbara, who does the pizza making, is cautiously starting to work on this method. She's now up to tossing it a mighty 4 or 5 inches.

Incidentally, if your pizza turns out to be oval or lopsided, don't let it bother you. In Italy, they sometimes make it that shape deliberately. It's called Pizza Rustica.

Okay, now it's on the peel. You may want to pinch up the edges a bit so your topping doesn't slide off when you shoot it into the oven. Put on the topping you select, open the oven door, and, with a shove forward and jerk back of the peel, shoot the pizza onto the stone or tiles. This sounds hard to do in contemplation, but it's really quite easy in execution.

How long do you bake your pizza? That pretty much depends on how hot your oven gets. It can range from 10 to 15 minutes. The best thing to do is just watch it. When the crust is golden brown, it's done. Slide your peel under the pizza and put the pizza on a round tray for serving and cutting with your roller-bladed pizza-cutting wheel. Cut each pizza into four servings.

4 slices Exchanges per serving: 1 starch Calories: 95
Protein: 2 gm Carbohydrate: 17 gm Fat: 2 gm Fiber: 0.5 gm
Cholesterol: 0 mg Sodium: 134 mg

(There is no way we can calculate whatever toppings you choose for your pizza; we trust you can estimate them yourselves.)

Toppings. As we pointed out above, when it comes to toppings you can put on just about anything you want. There are only a couple of restrictions. You don't want anything too wet, such as tomatoes that haven't had the seeds and juice squeezed out, or you'll make your beautiful crisp pizza into a soggy mess. You also don't want to put anything on the pizza that can't be cooked in around 15 minutes unless you cook it—or partially cook it—ahead of time.

To give you guidelines in choosing toppings, the following are some pizzas we serve when we're having our "panoply of pizzas" for guests.

Salmon Appetizer Pizza

Legend has it that Wolfgang Puck invented his salmon pizza once when, having no bagels on hand and seeking to appease someone wanting lox and bagels, he made a pizza and put the lox and sour cream on that. In our variation we make mini-pizzas by dividing the ball of dough into six parts and rolling each out and stretching it until it's about 2 to 2½ inches in diameter. Brush with olive oil. Put on a little finely chopped green onion or thinly sliced red onion. If you use the standard orange-colored smoked salmon (lox), cook the pizzas before you put it on. When possible, we prefer to use the smoked salmon from the Pacific Northwest that comes vacuum-packed in a foil pouch and needs no refrigeration. This is available by mail from two Seattle places: Pike Place Fish Market, (206) 682-7181; and City Fish Market, (206) 682-9329 (ask for David; his wife is diabetic, and he'll take particularly good care of you). When we use the Pacific Northwest variety of salmon we put it on the pizza before cooking, although it's already cooked.

When you take the pizzas out of the oven, garnish each with a dollop of low-fat sour cream with a little dill (preferably fresh) and a little ground pepper. If it's a really festive occasion, you can top it with a demitasse spoonful of caviar.

Caramelized Onions, Blue Cheese, and Rosemary Pizza

This is a variation on an Alice Waters recipe. We use much less onion (for diabetic purposes), and we're more flexible with the cheese: she specifies Gorgonzola, but it can just as well be blue cheese or Roquefort.

- 1 fairly large onion
- 1 teaspoon butter, margarine, or avocado oil
- 1 teaspoon olive oil
- 2 ounces blue cheese
- Rosemary
- Ground black pepper
- Pancetta (optional)

Slice the onion in the thinnest possible slices. Heat the butter, margarine, or avocado oil and the olive oil in a nonstick pan over the lowest heat. Add the onion and cook slowly, again on the lowest setting, until the onion is golden brown. (This may take as long as an hour. Just be sure the onion doesn't burn.)

When you're ready to make your pizza, spread the onions on the dough, dot the surface with blue cheese, and sprinkle with rosemary—preferably fresh. We go easy on the rosemary because many people aren't crazy about it and it can easily overwhelm the dish. When done, add a few coarse grindings of pepper. (When we feel we can afford the extra fat—which is seldom—we sometimes add a little pancetta, which we have cooked to the point of extreme crispiness in paper towels in the microwave.) We usually serve this with a green salad or a roasted-pepper salad.

Sun-Dried Tomatoes, Garlic, Black Olives, and Cheese Pizza

Sun-dried tomatoes are handy to have in the cupboard when tomatoes aren't at their best. They also deliver a good tomato flavor without excessive liquid. Reconstitute the tomatoes according to the directions on the package.

3 ounces low-fat mozzarella or dry Sonoma jack cheese
Chopped garlic
Sun dried tomatoes
5 or 10 black olives, Niçoise, Italian, or Greek

Grate the mozzarella or dry Sonoma jack cheese (California Gold Monterey Dry Jack, called *incomparable* by the *New York Times,* is similar in sharpness to a good moderately aged Parmesan; available from Vella Cheese Company, Box 191, Sonoma, CA 95476-0191; phone 1-800-848-0505), and sprinkle half of it on the pizza. Then top with a little chopped garlic, thin slices of the sun-dried tomatoes, and 5 big or 10 tiny chopped black olives of the Niçoise or Italian or Greek persuasion. (We use locally cured Niçoise ones that we get at the farmer's market.) Sprinkle with the rest of the cheese. Cook as usual, serve as usual, enjoy as usual.

As you can see, we make very light toppings. They're more subtle that way and you can use the pizza more like a bread course and serve it with a regular protein course. That way a diabetic can get enough protein. Of course, you can always put more protein on the pizza—such as sausage, ham, chicken, and so forth—and make it a main course. Aidel's Sausage Company of San Francisco makes an amazing variety of lower-fat sausages containing no MSG, binders, extenders, fillers, or preservatives except for the sodium nitrite required by law in smoked products. Call (415) 285-6660 for their tempting catalogue and recipes.

You can make calzone by putting your topping on only one half of the pizza dough and up to 1 inch from the edge, folding the unfilled side over, and, using a little water, pressing the edges together to seal. This puffs up beautifully in the oven.

You can also make great sandwich buns by dividing the ball of dough into thirds and rolling each third into a circle about 4½ inches in diameter. These, too, will puff up in the oven.

Pasta Perfect

Take a look at the "Pasta, Corn, Rice, Bread" section of the Glycemic Index and you'll see which has the lowest number: pasta. That gives us one more reason to love this versatile carbohydrate. Though we used to make fresh pasta, we find that now we're happy with any of the good imported Italian pastas (Agnesi, De Cecco, D'Aquino).

To cook pasta, always boil it in a large pot with preferably 12 cups of water, even though you're cooking just enough for one or two. A little olive oil helps keep things from sticking. Add 1 teaspoon of salt to the boiling water, unless you're sodium-restricted. You can used the instructions on the package as a guideline, but you must keep testing so you'll know the moment it's right. Fish out a strand, run it under cold water, and bite into it to see if it's *al dente*—tender but not mushily soft, firm but not with a hard, raw-tasting heart. (According to diabetes specialist Dr. Alan Marcus of South Orange County, California, "Overcooked pasta raises blood sugar because the boiling water changes the starch into sugar.") When it has reached this ephemeral state, remove it immediately, drain it, place it in a prewarmed bowl, and toss with the sauce, which you've had the foresight to make ahead of time. Get the pasta to the table as fast as you can and serve it in individual prewarmed bowls or plates. *One-half cup cooked pasta (1 ounce dry) is 1 Starch/Bread Exchange.*

The sauce on your pasta can be as simple as Olive Oil and Garlic Sauce, or Tomato Sauce, or it can be a more complex one such as Putanesca Sauce. Note: be sure not to drown the pasta in sauce; the sauce should just delicately coat the pasta the way salad dressing is supposed to just coat the greens.

Olive Oil and Garlic Sauce

Makes ½ cup sauce

- 2 teaspoons minced garlic
- ½ cup extra-virgin olive oil

for serving:

- 1 or 2 tablespoons of minced parsley
- Ground pepper

Sauté the minced garlic over low heat in the olive oil. Stirring it so it doesn't burn, cook the garlic until it becomes a rich, golden color. Toss this sauce with your *al dente* pasta, along with a tablespoon or two of minced parsley and a few grinds of pepper.

A one-tablespoon serving Exchanges per serving: 3 fat
Calories: 159 Protein: 0 gm Carbohydrate: 0 gm Fat: 18 gm
Fiber: 0 gm Cholesterol: 0 mg Sodium: 0 mg

Tomato Sauce

4 cups chopped tomatoes
1 tablespoon olive oil
1 finely chopped onion

Put the tomatoes—preferably homegrown or farmer's-market purchased—in a large bowl and pour boiling water over them to cover. After only a half minute, quickly take out the tomatoes with a slotted spoon and put them in a bowl of ice water (have a few cubes floating in the water). After another half minute remove from water and drain. Peel off the skin, slice the tomatoes across the middle (at the equator), and squeeze out the juice and seeds. Chop the tomatoes and, if they're still very juicy, drain in a colander or sieve. If you use canned tomatoes, get the Italian kind and drain off the liquid before chopping.

For every 4 cups of chopped tomatoes, sauté 1 finely chopped onion in 1 tablespoon olive oil, over low heat, covered, for around 10 minutes. Add the tomatoes and cook over higher heat, stirring constantly, for 5 to 10 minutes, or until most of the loose juice is gone. Process in a food processor. Use what you need and freeze the rest (it lasts 6 to 12 months).

½-cup serving Exchanges per serving: 1 vegetable Calories: 36
Protein: 1 gm Carbohydrate: 5 gm Fat: 2 gm Fiber: 1 gm
Cholesterol: 0 mg Sodium: 8 mg

You can make infinite variations on your tomato sauce by adding such things as herbs (fresh and dried), a couple of tablespoons of milk or cream, sautéed garlic, Parmesan cheese, and so forth. This sauce can be used on pizza as well as pasta, and it can be used as the base sauce even for non-Italian recipes.

Pasta Putanesca

Serves 4

- 2 cloves thinly sliced garlic
- 1½ tablespoons olive oil
- 3 anchovy fillets, or a 3-inch strip of anchovy paste
- 1 cup homemade tomato sauce, or 1 cup chopped canned Italian plum tomatoes
- 2½ teaspoons capers, rinsed and drained
- 6 Italian or Greek black olives, pitted and chopped
- 1 teaspoon chopped fresh parsley, or ½ teaspoon dried
- 1 teaspoon chopped fresh basil, or ½ teaspoon dried
- 1 teaspoon chopped fresh oregano, or ½ teaspoon dried
- Red pepper flakes to taste
- 8 ounces pasta

Sauté the garlic in olive oil until golden. Add the anchovy fillets that have been rinsed and mashed along with the homemade tomato sauce (or Italian plum tomatoes), the capers, the black olives (if you use the tiny French Niçoise olives, use 12), the fresh parsley, basil, and oregano, and the red-pepper flakes to taste. Simmer gently 10 to 15 minutes. Cook 8 ounces of pasta and toss with the sauce.

4 servings Exchanges per serving: 2 starch; ½ medium-fat meat; 1 fat; 1 vegetable Calories: 287 Protein: 9 gm Carbohydrate: 48 gm Fat: 7 gm Fiber: 5 gm Cholesterol: 0 mg Sodium: 94 mg

Your pasta becomes a main course with all the protein you need when you make the following:

Bolognese Sauce

Serves 4

- 2 tablespoons butter or margarine
- 2 tablespoons olive oil
- ½ cup finely chopped onion
- 2 tablespoons finely chopped carrot
- 2 tablespoons finely chopped celery
- ¾ pound ground lean beef
- ¾ pound ground turkey
- 1 cup dry white wine or white vermouth
- ½ cup nonfat milk
- 2 cups fresh tomatoes, or 2 cups chopped canned Italian plum tomatoes

serve with:
Grated Parmesan or Romano cheese

In a large, preferably enamel, pot or saucepan heat the butter or margarine and the olive oil. Add the onion, carrot, and celery. Sauté over medium heat until translucent and just barely starting to brown. Add the ground beef and ground turkey. Cook, stirring, until the meat loses its pink color. Add the white wine or white vermouth and cook over medium-high heat until the wine has evaporated. Add the milk and continue cooking until that has evaporated. Add the fresh tomatoes that have been peeled and seeded (see Tomato Sauce recipe) or canned tomatoes with their juice. Cover and, over low heat, simmer gently, stirring occasionally, for 2 hours, or until the sauce thickens. Rather than tossing the sauce with the pasta, put your pasta allotment in a heated bowl and top with your allotment of Bolognese Sauce. Sprinkle with grated Parmesan or Romano cheese.

½-cup serving Exchanges per serving: 2 medium-fat meat; 1 fat; ½ vegetable Calories: 192 Protein: 14 gm Carbohydrate: 3 gm Fat: 13 gm Fiber: 0.6 gm Cholesterol: 49 mg Sodium: 74 mg

Ravioli

An excellent way to create new and interesting dishes and even to use leftovers is to make ravioli. But we confess that until recently we found ravioli something of a chore to make, and they often turned out too thick and heavy. Finally, benevolent gods intervened and led us to an article in the February 1990 issue of *Gourmet* magazine. The title of the article was "Wonton Ravioli" and the author offered up the exciting idea that "wonton wrappers, stuffed and sealed, make perfect paper-thin ravioli." We raced out for a package of them—we got the round ones called Gyoza—and the good news turned out to be true!

We've been making and freezing quick and easy ravioli ever since. All you do is mix up your filling, put the wonton skin in the middle of a dumpling/ravioli maker (the same one we recommended for making potstickers), put 1 teaspoon of the filling in the middle of the wonton skin, brush the edges with beaten egg white, close the dumpling/ravioli maker firmly, open it, and there's your perfect ravioli (or would that be *raviolo?*). Keep them covered with a towel so they don't dry out. When you're ready, cook them in a large pot of gently boiling water, without crowding, for 2 minutes, or until they rise to the surface. As they are cooked, drain them on a paper towel and keep warm until you have all you need for that meal. Freeze the rest of the uncooked ravioli.

The *Gourmet* article featured some far-out but wonderful ravioli recipes such as Crab-Meat Ravioli with Fennel Purée and Roasted Red-Pepper Sauce; Corn, Pepper, and Monterey Jack Ravioli with Tomato Coriander Sauce; and Lamb and Spinach Ravioli with Minted Yogurt Sauce. (If you'd like to try some of these you can call 1-800-678-5681 and order a copy of the February 1990 issue of *Gourmet* for $4 plus $1.50 shipping.) But we're talking Italian here, folks, so for our ravioli you'll want to try some things like the following.

Chard (or Spinach) and Cheese Filling

Serves 7

- 3 tablespoons finely chopped onion
- 2 tablespoons vegetable oil or margarine
- 2 cups chopped cooked spinach or chard
- 1 cup ricotta
- 1 beaten egg white
- ½ cup grated Parmesan, Romano, or dry jack cheese
- ⅛ to ¼ teaspoon nutmeg

Sauté, until soft, the onion in vegetable oil or margarine. Add the spinach or chard, which you've squeezed all the moisture out of, and cook for 2 minutes. In a mixing bowl combine the spinach or chard mixture with the ricotta, beaten egg white, grated cheese, and nutmeg.

7 servings Exchanges per serving of 4 ravioli: 1 starch; 1 medium-fat meat; 1 fat; ½ vegetable Calories: 212 Protein: 9 gm Carbohydrate: 24 gm Fat: 9 gm Fiber: 1 gm Cholesterol: 16 mg Sodium: 221 mg

Meat Filling

- 2 cups ground cooked beef, pork, chicken, or turkey
- 3 tablespoons finely chopped onion
- 1 clove finely chopped garlic
- 2 tablespoons olive or vegetable oil
- 2 tablespoons finely chopped parsley
- 1 beaten egg white
- ¼ cup grated cheese
- Salt to taste (optional)
- Freshly ground pepper to taste

Begin with 2 cups of any one or a combination: ground cooked meat. (Use leftovers when you can.) Cook the onion and garlic in the olive or vegetable oil until the onion and garlic are soft but not brown. Add the ground meat and cook, stirring, for 1 minute. Remove from the heat and mix in the parsley, egg white, cheese, salt (optional), and freshly ground pepper to taste.

7 servings Exchanges per serving of 4 ravioli: 1 starch; 2 medium-fat meat; 1 fat Calories: 277 Protein: 16 gm Carbohydrate: 21 gm Fat: 14 gm Fiber: 0 gm Cholesterol: 109 mg Sodium: 51 mg

Sweet-Potato Filling

Serves 6–7

- 1¾ pounds cooked sweet potatoes, pureed
- ½ cup grated cheese
- 3 tablespoons finely chopped parsley
- 2 tablespoons chopped ham, preferably prosciutto (optional)
- 2 beaten egg whites
- ¼ to ½ teaspoon nutmeg
- Salt to taste (optional)

Combine the cooked sweet potatoes, which you have pureed in a food processor until smooth, with the grated cheese, finely chopped parsley, chopped ham, beaten egg whites, nutmeg, and salt to taste (also optional). Mix thoroughly.

6 to 7 servings Exchanges per serving of 4 ravioli: 1 starch; 1 medium-fat meat Calories: 239 Protein: 7 gm Carbohydrate: 46 gm Fat: 3 gm Fiber: 2 gm Cholesterol: 7 mg Sodium: 264 mg

Sauces for Ravioli

Use anything you like: just a little butter or margarine and grated cheese, Tomato Sauce (with or without added herbs),

Tomato Sauce smoothed out with a little milk, Bolognese Sauce (don't use with meat ravioli as that would be not only redundant but also boring), pesto sauce (blend 1 cup fresh basil, 1/4 cup olive oil, 1 tablespoon pine nuts, 1 large clove garlic, and 3 to 4 tablespoons grated cheese), and anything else your active imagination dictates.

Risotto. To our minds, risotto is the most wonderfully rich and creamy of all the world's rice dishes. The most praised of all Italian cookbook authors, Marcella Hazan, calls risotto "a uniquely Italian technique for cooking rice . . . almost a cuisine all by itself." We can only share with you here its most famous form, Risotto alla Milanese (risotto in the Milan style) and one variation, plus a few ideas for others. Risotto should be made with unwashed Arborio rice from northern Italy. (California's short-grained pearl rice is okay, too.)

The method for cooking risotto differs from all other rice-cooking methods in that the liquid is added a small amount at a time. It is truly a handcrafted dish in the sense that you stand and stir for at least 20 minutes until the rice becomes, in Hazan's words, "a creamy union of tender, yet firm grains." But we find that risotto can be made quickly, easily, and reliably in the microwave. The secret is to cook the rice for a total of only about 18 minutes, stirring only two or three times.

Risotto alla Milanese

Serves 4

- 1 small onion, minced
- 3 tablespoons butter or avocado oil
- 1 cup Arborio rice
- 1 cup chicken stock
- 1 cup dry white wine
- Dash ground saffron

for serving:

- 1/3 cup finely grated Parmesan cheese
- Salt and pepper to taste

Combine the onion with the butter (or avocado oil) in a 2½-quart microwave casserole dish. Cover with wax paper and microwave on high for about 3 minutes, or until the onion is translucent. Mix in the rice, cover with wax paper, and microwave on high for 1 minute. Mix together chicken stock, white wine, and a dash of ground saffron. Add to rice, cover with a tight lid, and microwave on high for 5 to 7 minutes, or until boiling. Stir. Put the lid on and microwave on medium for 9 to 10 minutes, or until almost all the liquid is absorbed and the rice tastes *al dente* (firm to the bite). Cover again and let stand 5 minutes. Just before serving, take a fork and stir in Parmesan cheese; add salt and pepper to taste.

4 servings Exchanges per serving: 2 starch; ½ medium-fat meat; 2 fat Calories: 290 Protein: 7 gm Carbohydrate: 39 gm Fat: 11 gm Fiber: 1 gm Cholesterol: 30 mg Sodium: 246 mg

Windsor's White-Wine Risotto

Serves 6

We've tried several microwave recipes, but find that this one, courtesy of Windsor Vineyards of California, is the best. We particularly like it with peeled and seeded tomatoes we've just picked out of our own yard, instead of the canned ones.

½ cup olive oil
½ medium onion, chopped
2 cloves garlic, chopped
1½ cups Arborio rice
1½ cups chicken broth
½ cup white wine
Juice of half a lemon
1 8-ounce can Italian plum tomatoes, drained

to serve:
½ cup grated Parmesan cheese

Heat the olive oil in a skillet and sauté the onion and garlic. Add the rice, stirring until the rice grains turn opaque. Mix the chicken broth with white wine and lemon juice in a measuring cup. Then pour the contents of the skillet into a large microwave casserole dish with a top, adding the tomatoes. Add one-third of the liquid mixture from the measuring cup. Put the top on the casserole dish and cook in the microwave at high for 5 minutes.

Remove the dish and stir gently so that no rice is sticking to the bottom. Then add another third of the liquid and cook on high for 5 more minutes. Remove from the microwave and stir, adding the rest of the liquid, and microwave for 5 more minutes. Remove and stir a third time. The rice should be creamy, with a small amount of liquid. Stir in Parmesan cheese and serve.

6 servings Exchanges per serving: 2 starch; 3½ fat; ½ medium-fat meat; ½ vegetable Calories: 380 Protein: 7 gm Carbohydrate: 40 gm Fat: 20 gm Fiber: 1 gm Cholesterol: 6 mg Sodium: 220 mg

Other Ideas

With fresh mushrooms. Sauté about 4 ounces of mushrooms in oil or butter. Proceed with the Risotto alla Milanese recipe, adding the mushrooms at the end, when you add the cheese.

With dried porcini mushrooms. Soak ½ ounce porcini mushrooms in warm water for 20 minutes; drain, rinse, and squeeze. Reserve the liquid and substitute it for part of the chicken stock in either risotto recipe (a little goes a long way). Add the mushrooms as above.

Asparagus, peas, spinach, or zucchini can also be used. Usually the vegetables are cooked first and added at either the beginning or the end. For guidance it's best to consult a good Italian cookbook—our current favorite being *Northern Italian Cooking* by Biba Caggiano (HP Books). Biba is the owner and chef of an outstanding restaurant in Sacramento, the eponymous (we've always wanted to use that word!) Biba's. Under her gentle guidance, you may even want to venture making risotto the classic way. And you certainly should try her other wonderful recipes. We particularly recommend her stuffed chicken breasts (slightly modified for the diabetic diet).

Stuffed Chicken Breasts Biba

Serves 6

- 3 whole chicken breasts
- 3 paper-thin slices Prosciutto
- 3 thin slices fontina or 3 tablespoons Parmesan cheese
- 1½ sage leaves
- Milk
- Flour
- 3 tablespoons butter or margarine
- 1 tablespoon olive oil
- 1 crushed chicken bouillon cube
- 1 cup dry white wine *in all*
- Salt (optional)
- Freshly ground pepper to taste
- ⅓ cup whipping cream, whole milk, or nonfat milk

Skin, bone, and split the chicken breasts. Put a slice of prosciutto, a slice of fontina, or a tablespoon of Parmesan cheese, and half a sage leaf on each breast. Roll up the breasts and secure them with wooden toothpicks. Dip them in milk, then roll in flour to lightly coat. Melt the butter or margarine in the olive oil. When butter or margarine foams, add the chicken breasts. Cook over medium heat until golden on all sides. Add the crushed chicken bouillon cube and ½ cup of the white wine. Add salt (optional) and freshly ground pepper to taste. When wine is reduced by half, add the remaining white wine. Cover skillet and reduce heat. Simmer 15 to 20 minutes, or until chicken is tender. Turn chicken several times during cooking. Add a little more wine if the sauce looks too dry.

Place chicken on a warm platter. Increase heat and add the whipping cream, milk, or nonfat milk (depending on how many Fat Exchanges you can afford to use). Deglaze the skillet by stirring to dissolve meat juices attached to the bottom. Taste the sauce and adjust the seasoning; then spoon it over the chicken. Serve immediately.

6 servings Exchanges per serving: 2 medium-fat meat; 2 fat
Calories: 271 Protein: 28 gm Carbohydrate: 0.5 gm
Fat: 15 gm Fiber: 0 gm Cholesterol: 102 mg Sodium: 198 mg

Finishing our Italian adventure on this culinary high point, we wish you *buon apetito e buona vita!*

DESSERTS
SWEET SOMETHINGS

Desserts are notorious comfort foods. (That's what gets people into so much trouble with them!) Although we usually find our food comforts elsewhere, we always serve them to guests. And June usually plays dessert chef since in that way she has total control over content and portion size. Here are desserts she particularly enjoys making—and eating—and so do our guests.

Rice Pudding

Serves 6

The Grill on the Alley, a posh Beverly Hills restaurant near Rodeo Drive, has created Southern California's most popular rice pudding, and we've finally perfected our own diabetic version of it. Barbara likes it for breakfast and June likes it for lunch or a snack, and everybody likes it for dinner dessert. To escalate this pudding into the realm of the exotic, use perfumy Indian basmati rice instead of ordinary white rice.

- 1/4 cup raisins
- 1 tablespoon butter
- 3½ cups milk
- ½ cup white rice
- 1 ½-inch piece of vanilla bean
- 1 cinnamon stick
- 4 packets of Sweet One
- 1 egg yolk
- 2 tablespoons water

First boil the raisins for 3 minutes in water to cover. Allow these to cool while you're doing the rest. In a one-gallon saucepan put the butter, milk, rice, the piece of vanilla bean, cinnamon stick, and packets of Sweet One. Bring to a boil and simmer 8 minutes, stirring every 2 or 3 minutes. Then beat the egg yolk with 2 tablespoons water and stir this into the rice. Simmer 10 minutes longer, stirring occasionally. Remove the vanilla bean and cinnamon stick and put the pudding into a refrigerator container, add the drained raisins, and refrigerate for 2 to 3 hours. Serve in half-cup containers, garnished with cinnamon.

6 servings Exchanges per serving: ½ starch; ½ medium-fat meat; ⅓ fruit Calories: 139 Protein: 6 gm Carbohydrate: 21 gm Fat: 3 gm Fiber: 0.5 gm Cholesterol: 43 mg Sodium: 96 mg

Not-So-Naughty Mud Cake

Serves 8

Those of you who've traveled to the island of Kauai may have seen a diabetically sinful dessert called Naughty Hula Pie on the menu at the Kiahuna Plantation restaurant. Our mud cake is not so naughty as that, but it is a close relative and to be used only as a rare treat. Its fat content is beyond redemption, so we don't even try to do a modified version except for using fructose instead of sugar.

We discovered this recipe through Ruth Reichl, food editor of the Los Angeles Times, *who in turn got it from the* Fanny Farmer Baking Book. *Here's her description of it: "This cake is about as easy as a cake can be. You can mix the batter right in the pan that you melt the chocolate in, so there's no bowl to wash. The cake needs no frosting. Best of all, it tastes completely wonderful. It's dark and dense, with a sophisticated flavor that no mix ever had."*

- 4 one-ounce squares unsweetened chocolate
- 6 tablespoons butter
- ¾ cup strong-brewed coffee
- 2 tablespoons bourbon
- 2 eggs
- ½ teaspoon vanilla extract
- 1¼ cups cake flour
- ½ cup granular fructose
- ½ teaspoon baking soda
- ⅛ teaspoon salt

serve with:
Vanilla ice cream or unsweetened whipped cream

Combine the unsweetened chocolate, butter, and coffee in a heavy saucepan. Heat over very low heat until the chocolate melts, stirring until smooth and blended. Cool 10 minutes. Beat in the bourbon, eggs, and vanilla extract.

Sift the cake flour with the fructose, baking soda, and salt. Add to chocolate mixture, beating until smooth. Pour into a greased and floured 8-by-4-inch loaf pan. Bake at 275 degrees for 45 to 55 minutes. Cool in the pan for 15 minutes, then turn out onto a rack and allow to cool completely.

Serve with a vanilla ice cream or a tiny bit of unsweetened whipped cream.

8 servings Exchanges per serving: 1 starch; 1½ fat; ⅓ milk
Calories: 202 Protein: 4 gm Carbohydrate: 34 gm
Fat: 6 gm Fiber: 1 gm Cholesterol: 103 mg Sodium: 103 mg

Sweet Potatoes Dulles

Serves 6

Our name for this dessert comes from where we discovered it: the Hyatt Hotel at Dulles Airport, where we spent the night prior to taking an early-morning flight.

This unusual dessert actually wasn't planned as a dessert. It was a side dish served with one of the main courses. Since it was made with sweet potatoes, which occupy a place much lower on the Glycemic Index than you would expect considering their sweet taste, we wanted to try it, but it wasn't served as part of either main course we were ordering. The amiable waitress was kind enough to make a substitution for us so we could have a taste. With the first bite we realized that with minor adjustments it would make a fabulous dessert. The chef was kind enough to write up the recipe for us. We use Fruit Sweet (see the recipe below) instead of honey and condensed nonfat milk instead of cream, but we think it tastes just as great as the original.

- 1 cup cooked sweet potatoes
- 1 egg
- 2 egg whites
- 1 cup condensed nonfat milk
- 1/8 teaspoon salt
- 3 tablespoons Fruit Sweet
- 1 teaspoon cinnamon (or to taste)

serve with:
Yoghurt or sugar-free whipped topping

In a food processor, combine the sweet potatoes with the whole egg and egg whites and process until smooth. Place this puree in a bowl and whisk in the condensed milk, salt, Fruit Sweet (available from Wax Orchards; call 1-800-634-6132), and cinnamon.

Preheat the oven to 325 degrees. Spray thoroughly 6 small ramekins or custard cups with Pam and fill 3/4 full with the potato batter. Place the cups in an ovenproof pan and add hot water to the pan to a level halfway up the cups. Bake for 35 to

40 minutes, or until a knife inserted in the potatoes comes out clean.

Either serve in the cups or turn them upside down on a plate. (You may have to put the cups in hot water and/or run a knife blade around the outside edge to loosen the potatoes.) Sweet Potatoes Dulles is delicious by itself, or you can top it off with a little yoghurt or sugar-free whipped topping.

6 servings Exchanges per serving: ½ starch; ½ milk Calories: 105 Protein: 6 gm Carbohydrate: 18 gm Fat: 1 gm Fiber: 1 gm Cholesterol: 37 mg Sodium: 154 mg

And now we need a little bistro dessert. We'll make it light, we'll make it . . .

Pears Amandine

Serves 6

- 1 cup water
- 2 or 3 drops vanilla extract or 1 inch of vanilla bean
- 3 packets of Sweet One
- 3 fresh, ripe, but firm pears
- 1 cup sliced strawberries
- 2 or 3 slivers of toasted almond

Boil the water to which you've added the vanilla extract or vanilla bean and the packets of Sweet One. In this mixture poach for 8 minutes the pears, halved and cored. Remove the pears and place, flat side down, on a plate to cool.

Reduce the poaching syrup by simmering down to about ½ cup. Add the strawberries and boil until you have a nice syrupy syrup. Pour into the blender or food processor and whirl until smooth. Stick a few slivers of toasted almond into each pear half and spoon some strawberry sauce over it. Refrigerate until serving time.

6 servings Exchanges per serving: 1 fruit Calories: 56
Protein: 0.5 gm Carbohydrate: 14 gm Fat: 0.5 gm Fiber: 3 gm
Cholesterol: 0 mg Sodium: 1 mg

If you want to step a bit off the fruit route, cover poached pears with Fudge Sweet (available from Wax Orchards; call 1-800-634-6132).

Afterword: You and Your Doctor

Although we've repeatedly pointed out that your diabetes control and your total health are primarily your responsibility, you can't do it alone. For the best therapy you need the help of a whole team of dedicated diabetes health professionals, and your co-captain of that team is your physician. Since diabetics work more closely (and longer!) with their doctors, they need to be particularly certain that they have just the right one.

If you have any doubts about the kind of care you're getting from your doctor, you might look over these twelve warning signs. They're from the book *Playing God: The New World of Medical Choices* by Drs. Thomas Scully and Celia Scully. They seem to us to be especially significant for diabetics.

Clues You're Not Getting the Care You Should*

Your doctor:

1. Doesn't seem to be listening to what you are telling him or her.
2. Doesn't answer your questions or take time to ask if you have any. When an answer is given, it is in words you don't understand.

*Reprinted from *Playing God: The New World of Medical Choices* by Thomas Scully and Celia Scully (New York: Simon and Schuster, 1987, pp. 43–44).

3. Fails to take an adequate medical history or give you a complete physical examination when it is called for.
4. Doesn't help you learn more about your condition and what you can do about it, and gives no explanation as to why the recommended tests, treatment, or medications might be necessary.
5. Neglects to inform you of potential risks, benefits, and side effects of prescribed drugs or suggested procedures and tests. (Beware if you have told your physician that you are allergic to a certain medication and it is prescribed anyway.)
6. (*for women*) Doesn't respect your modesty and makes suggestive remarks while doing a pelvic examination or examining your breasts.
7. Fails to make a follow-up appointment for you and does not instruct you to call the office to report on how you are doing.
8. Seems forgetful, peculiar, or belligerent, or has alcohol on his or her breath.
9. Is hard to reach, doesn't return phone calls, and fails to arrange for another doctor to care for you when he or she is out of town.
10. Is not on the staff of any community hospital or medical center.
11. Is rigid, acts as if he or she knows it all, and insists that the only way to treat your condition is his or her way.
12. Reacts defensively when you suggest a second opinion.

Another warning signal we might add is if your doctor doesn't practice *preventive* medicine.

The *First Surgeon General's Report on Health Promotion and Disease Prevention* declares that "prevention is a health idea whose time has come." We echo that declaration and, strangely enough, while we were formulating our own ideas on preventing diabetes problems through a total-health program June received this letter from her doctor.

Dear Patients:

We would like to tell you of a shift in the emphasis in our practice. This change will be gradual and will not jeopardize our individual relationships with our patients, but should enhance the existing personalized treatment.

For many years our primary interest in medicine has been the prevention and treatment of cardiovascular disease and diabetes, particularly coronary disease, high blood pressure, heart attack, and stroke. Clinical research now available, in combination with our experience of the last thirty years, has produced convincing evidence that it is possible to detect and recognize certain Risk Factors which are often associated with these diseases. Fortunately, many of these Risk Factors can be altered favorably by the proper use of diet, medication, and healthful changes in habits and lifestyle. Proper control of these Risk Factors may prevent, defer, or ameliorate these diseases.

The most important Risk Factors which *can* be influenced favorably are *high blood pressure, cigarette smoking, high blood fats* (cholesterol, triglycerides, lipoproteins), and *diabetes.* Other Risk Factors which can be treated are *obesity, excessive stress,* and *lack of proper exercise.*

Risk Factor Reduction offers the greatest promise in the prevention of cardiovascular disease and diabetes. Our practice in the future will stress preventive medicine through Risk Factor Detection and Reduction in an integrated program for all our patients.

In the field of diagnosis more time will be spent on very detailed history-taking and physical examination. Laboratory studies will include, in addition to the usual studies, treadmill stress tests, blood-lipid studies, and appropriate cardiac monitoring. Further diagnostic tests will be done where indicated.

After completion of these studies, a personal conference will be arranged to discuss, in detail, results and diagnoses and to give careful instructions concerning medications, diet, exercise, and other aspects of lifestyle. With our active cooperation and participation, patients will be deeply involved in assuming more responsibility for their own health. Periodic check-ups will be performed to evaluate individual progress.

The prevention and treatment of cardiovascular disease and diabetes are most effective if begun early in one's life. Therefore new patients entering our practice will generally be under the age of fifty.

Patients of all ages who are already in our practice have our assurance that we will continue to care for them as in the past with even greater attention to our philosophy of Risk Factor Detection and Reduction. As always, if an emergency medical problem should arise, our office will be available for appropriate care and advice.

We will be of greater service to our patients by this expanded approach in our practice of Cardiology and Internal Medicine.

If you have any questions or comments we would like very much to hear from you.

It's almost like the invention of radar—several people working out the same good idea independently and announcing their discoveries almost simultaneously.

There are a number of other health-radar inventors operating at this point in health time. Possibly the biggest breakthroughs are coming in the live-in health-enhancement centers where you and members of your family come to learn to change your whole lifestyle. Although centers of this sort are springing up all across the nation, we seem to have a fairly large number of them in the Southern California area. One of these is the Center for Health Enhancement Education and Research (CHEER) at UCLA. To give you an idea of what such centers do for you, these are excerpts from the CHEER brochure:

A Four-Week Intensive Course in Wellness, Health Enhancement, and Lifestyle Change

Teaching "wellness."

Teaching people to take responsibility for their own health. Focusing on the reduction and prevention of hypertension (high blood pressure), obesity, blood fats, smoking, and diabetes mellitus, which contribute so greatly to coronary or atherosclerotic heart disease, "hardening of the arteries," and other diseases of the blood vessels including those that lead to stroke and chronic lung, liver, eye, and kidney diseases.

Helping people adopt new health habits and lifestyles.

Offering long-term follow-up support for participants, their spouses, and their families.

When you enroll in the program, the CHEER senior staff, all faculty members of the Schools of Medicine and Public Health, will prepare a complete health profile for you. It will be based on information obtained through preliminary consultation with your physician and from CHEER's own thorough physical, laboratory, and psychosocial examinations. You will then receive a prescribed plan of diet, exercise, and psychosocial consultation, and while you are working through your program many of the physical and lab tests will be repeated at weekly intervals in order to determine your progress in an objective way.

All exercise programs will be under the supervision of members of the UCLA faculty. After you have undergone continuous, electronically monitored stress testing on a treadmill, CHEER staff will "tailor" a program of exercise to your individual needs, your capacity, and your previous exercise habits. Together with the other CHEER participants, you will enjoy three appetizing and healthy meals a day, plus midmorning and evening snacks prepared in "gourmet" health cooking fashion under the supervision of the CHEER nutritionist-dietitian.

Interspersed with meals and exercise hours will be several hours daily of lectures, workshops, and group discussions on such topics as *Nutritional Fads and Fallacies, How to Maintain a CHEER Diet and Enjoy Eating Out, Sex and the Coronary Patient, Cardiovascular Disease and Exercise, Relaxation Techniques, Practice Cooking Sessions,* and *How to Live with CHEER in the Home.*

Centers like this provide a wonderful learning experience provided you have the time and the money (around $4,000) to spare. Indeed, investing that much in a program sometimes makes a person take the advice more seriously.

We believe, however, that by using this book and working closely with your own doctor and other diabetes health-care professionals you can create your own health-enhancement program and do it in the area in which you're going to be practicing it—your own environment and your own daily life.

A survey by Louis Harris showed that a majority of Americans would like their doctors to advise them on preventive health measures but that only a small minority of doctors do so. We don't blame the doctors for this. We say, along with the warden in the film *Cool Hand Luke,* "What we have here is a failure to communicate." Probably that majority of Americans never *tell* the doctor they'd like advice on preventive health measures. We think that if you do tell your doctor you'll get nothing but enthusiastic cooperation. (You might even show him or her June's doctor's letter.)

As part of your prevention program with your doctor we think you should have an understanding program. That is to say, we think you should ask for a full explanation of all test results. For example, you shouldn't just know that your blood sugar is "okay" or your cholesterol is "average for your age" or your triglycerides are "a little on the high side." You should know the exact numbers and understand their significance. (This also gives you a basis for comparison for the future improvement you're bound to have with your new lifestyle.) In explaining these figures and other aspects of your health to you, your doctor needs to become as much a teacher as a healer. Barbara Brown, the biofeedback expert, warns that this is the hardest shift for some doctors to make, because it is a new role for them. But we feel that when they do learn to share their knowledge and the responsibility for your good health with you, both of you will gain.

We also think you should ask your doctor to recommend a dietitian if there isn't one on staff. You should work with this dietitian on planning your individual diet, especially if you intend to make any deviations from the standard Exchange Lists. In our opinion, a dietitian is one of the most vital (and unfortunately one of the most frequently missing) members of your total-health-program team. Most doctors have neither the time, the inclination, nor the background to give you the individual dietary counseling you need to bring about optimum health and control.

If your doctor doesn't have the name of a dietitian for you, call your local hospital and ask the dietitian there for a referral, or write the American Dietetic Association, 430 North Michigan Avenue, Chicago, IL 60611.

Another thing we heartily recommend is taking a diabetes-education course. Most of these are reasonably priced and some are even free. At these courses you receive instruction from doctors, nurses, and dietitians and sometimes from social workers, psychologists, and exercise therapists. Call your local diabetes association to find out what courses are available in your area or write or call the American Association of Diabetes Educators, 444 North Michigan Avenue, Suite 1240, Chicago, IL 60611; phone 1-800-338-DMED.

Get busy working out your prevention program. Do it now! The life you enhance and prolong will definitely be your own.

APPENDIX A
Bernstein's Chart of Food Conversion to Glucose

Food Type and Conversion Process	Approximate Timing for Digestion, Conversion to Glucose, and Appearance as Increased BG: BG Rise Begins	Last Trace of Glucose Appears in Blood
Glucose. No digestion required. Moves directly through stomach and intestinal walls into bloodstream.	2 minutes	½ hour
Fructose (fruit sugar). No digestion required. Moves into blood-stream through intestinal walls. Converted by liver to triose-phosphates, which also are intermediate products of glucose metabolism. These will convert to glucose if not covered by additional insulin.	25 minutes	1½ hours
Sugar alcohols (used as artificial sweeteners, also found in fruits and vegetables). Converted in a manner similar to fructose.	25 minutes	1½ hours
Sucrose (table sugar). Digestion breaks the glucose molecule away from the fructose molecule. The two separate molecules then proceed as above with the original glucose portion appearing as BG first.	5 minutes	1½ hours
Starch and other polysaccharides. Salivary (and pancreatic) amylase breaks down much of it to maltose, which is further degraded to glucose in the small intestine.	10 minutes	1½ hours
Protein. Denatured by acids in stomach, then broken down into amino acids by digestive enzymes in small intestine. Amino acids enter bloodstream and those not used for tissue building are converted to glucose by the liver.	1½ hours (If we ignore the Phase I glucagon effect that can be offset by relatively low blood levels of insulin)	4 hours
Fat. Is not converted to glucose. There does exist a Phase I glucagon effect if consumed in large amounts. This can be offset by relatively low blood levels of insulin.		

Reprinted by permission from *Diabetes: The GlucoGraf Method for Normalizing Blood Sugar* by Richard K. Bernstein (Los Angeles, Jeremy P. Tarcher, Inc., 1983).

APPENDIX B

Glycemic Index

The Glycemic Index is basically a classification of how high and how fast the blood sugar is raised by individual carbohydrate foods. The index compares the way carbohydrate foods raise blood sugar with the way straight glucose raises it. Glucose, the form of sugar in the blood, is assigned an index number of 100.

Generally speaking, for a diabetic a low (slow-releasing) Glycemic Index food is preferred to a high (fast-releasing) Glycemic Index food. The chart on the following two pages shows the Glycemic Index of some foods that have been tested.

Simple Sugars

Fructose—20	Honey—87
Sucrose—59	Glucose—100

Fruits

Apples—39	Bananas—62
Oranges—40	Raisins—64
Orange juice—48	

Starchy Vegetables

Sweet potatoes—48	Instant potatoes—80
Yams—51	Carrots—92
Beets—64	Parsnips—97
White potatoes—70	

Dairy Products

Skim milk—32	Ice cream—36
Whole milk—34	Yogurt—36

Legumes

Soybeans—15	Garbanzos—36
Lentils—29	Lima beans—36
Kidney beans—29	Baked beans—40
Black-eyed peas—33	Frozen peas—51

Pasta, Corn, Rice, Bread

Whole-wheat pasta—42	White bread—69
White pasta—50	Whole-wheat bread—72
Sweet corn—59	White rice—72
Brown rice—66	

Breakfast Cereals

Oatmeal—49	Shredded wheat—67
All-Bran—51	Cornflakes—80
Swiss Muesli—66	

Miscellaneous

Peanuts—13	Sponge cake—46
Sausages—28	Potato chips—51
Fish sticks—38	Mars bars—68
Tomato soup—38	

APPENDIX C

Chart of Calorie Expenditures

	Gross Energy Cost (calories per hour)
Rest and Light Activity	**50–200**
Lying down or sleeping	80
Sitting	100
Driving an automobile	120
Standing	140
Domestic work	180
Moderate Activity	**200–350**
Bicycling (5½ mph)	210
Walking (2½ mph)	210
Gardening	220
Canoeing (2½ mph)	230
Golf	250
Lawn mowing (power mower)	250
Bowling	270
Lawn mowing (hand mower)	270
Fencing	300
Rowboating (2½ mph)	300
Swimming (¼ mph)	300
Walking (3¾ mph)	300
Badminton	350
Horseback riding (trotting)	350
Square dancing	350
Volleyball	350
Roller skating	350

Vigorous Activity	**over 350**
Table tennis	360
Ditch digging (hand shovel)	400
Ice skating (10 mph)	400
Wood chopping or sawing	400
Tennis	420
Waterskiing	480
Hill climbing (100 ft. per hr.)	490
Skiing (10 mph)	600
Squash and handball	600
Cycling (13 mph)	660
Scull rowing (race)	840
Running (10 mph)	900

Reprinted from *The Diabetic's Sports and Exercise Book* by June Biermann and Barbara Toohey (Philadelphia, J. B. Lippincott, 1977).

Suggested Reading

A STRONG BODY

Anderson, James W. *HCF Guide Book.* Lexington, KY: HCF Diabetes Research Foundation, 1987.

Anderson, James W., et al. *HCF Exchanges.* Lexington, KY: HCF Diabetes Research Foundation, 1987.

Bernstein, Richard K. *Diabetes: The GlucoGraf Method for Normalizing Blood Sugar.* Los Angeles: Jeremy P. Tarcher, 1983.

______. *Diabetes Type II.* New York: Prentice-Hall, 1990.

Bienefeld, Florence, and Bienefeld, Mickey. *The Vegetarian Gourmet.* Beverly Hills: Royal House Publishing, 1987.

Biermann, June, and Toohey, Barbara. *The Diabetic's Book: All Your Questions Answered.* Revised Edition. Los Angeles: Jeremy P. Tarcher, 1990.

______. *The Diabetic's Sports and Exercise Book.* New York: Lippincott, 1977.

Editors of Sunset Books and Magazines. *Sunset Vegetarian Cooking.* Menlo Park, CA: Sunset Publishing Company, 1981.

Exchange Lists for Meal Planning. Alexandria, VA: American Diabetes Association, 1986.

Fleck, S. J., and Kraemer, W. J. *Designing Resistance Training Programs.* Champaigne, IL: Human Kinetics Books, 1987.

Franz, Marion J. *Exchanges for All Occasions.* Wayzata, MN: Diabetes Centers, 1987.

Jovanovic, Lois; Biermann, June; and Toohey, Barbara. *The Diabetic Woman.* Los Angeles: Jeremy P. Tarcher, 1987.

Lodewick, Peter; Biermann, June; and Toohey, Barbara. *The Diabetic Man.* Los Angeles: Lowell House, 1991.

Robertson, Laurel; Flinders, Carol; and Godfrey, Bronwen. *The New Laurel's Kitchen.* Berkeley, CA: Ten Speed Press, 1986.

Scully, Thomas, and Scully, Celia. *Playing God: The New World of Medical Choices.* New York: Simon and Schuster, 1987.

Stout, Ruth, and Clemence, Richard. *The No-Work Garden Book.* Emmaus, PA: Rodale Press, 1971.

Thomas, Anna. *The Vegetarian Epicure.* New York: Vintage Books, 1972.

———. *The Vegetarian Epicure: Book Two.* New York: Knopf, 1978.

Todd, Jerry, and Todd, Jan. *Lift Your Way to Youthful Fitness.* Boston: Little, Brown, 1985.

Westcott, Wayne. *Building Strength at the YMCA.* Champaigne, IL: Human Kinetics Books, 1987.

A TRANQUIL MIND

Benson, Herbert, and Klipper, Miriam A. *The Relaxation Response.* New York: Avon Books, 1976.

Borysenko, Joan. *Minding the Body, Mending the Mind.* Reading, MA: Addison Wesley, 1978.

Jacobson, Edmond. *Progressive Relaxation.* Chicago: University of Chicago Press, 1938.

LeShan, Lawrence. *How to Meditate.* New York: Bantam Books, 1984.

Lindemann, Hannes. *Relieve Tension the Autogenic Way.* New York: P. H. Wyden, 1973.

Siegel, Bernie S. *Peace, Love and Healing.* New York: Harper and Row, 1989.

A BLITHE SPIRIT

Biermann, June, and Toohey, Barbara. *The Peripatetic Diabetic.* Revised Edition. Los Angeles: Jeremy P. Tarcher, 1983.

______. *Personhood: The Art of Being Fully Human.* New York: Fawcett Columbine, 1978.

______. *Bus 9 to Paradise.* New York: Fawcett Columbine, 1986.

Buscaglia, Leo. *Love.* New York: Fawcett Crest, 1972.

Colton, Helen. *The Joy of Touching.* New York: Simon and Schuster, 1980.

Moody, Raymond A. *Laugh after Laugh: The Healing Power of Humor.* Jackson, FL: Headwaters Press, 1978.

AN ECLECTIC COOKBOOK FOR DIABETICS

Caggiano, Biba. *Northern Italian Cooking.* Los Angeles: HP Books, 1981.

Editors of Sunset Books and Magazines. *The Sunset Stir-Fry Cookbook.* Menlo Park, CA: Sunset Publishing Company, 1988.

BOOK SOURCE

New books on diabetes and related total health topics are continually being published. If you would like a free copy of *The Diabetic Reader,* a newsletter that reviews the best of these, please write to us: Barbara Toohey and June Biermann, 5623 Matilija Avenue, Van Nuys, CA 91401; or call, 1-800-735-7726.

Index